End Back & Neck Pain

Vincent Fortanasce, MD

David Gutkind, DPT

Robert G. Watkins, III, MD

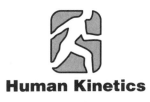

Human Kinetics

Library of Congress Cataloging-in-Publication Data

Fortanasce, Vincent.
  End back & neck pain / Vincent Fortanasce, David Gutkind, Robert G. Watkins, III.
    p. cm.
  Includes index.
  ISBN-13: 978-0-7360-9528-0 (soft cover)
  ISBN-10: 0-7360-9528-4 (soft cover)
  1. Backache--Treatment. 2. Neck pain--Treatment. 3. Self-care, Health. I. Gutkind, David, 1964-
II. Watkins, Robert G. III. Title. IV. Title: End back and neck pain.
  RD771.B217F67 2012
  617.5'64--dc23

                                    2011017968

ISBN-10: 0-7360-9528-4 (print)
ISBN-13: 978-0-7360-9528-0 (print)

This publication is written and published to provide accurate and authoritative information relevant to the subject matter presented. It is published and sold with the understanding that the author and publisher are not engaged in rendering legal, medical, or other professional services by reason of their authorship or publication of this work. If medical or other expert assistance is required, the services of a competent professional person should be sought.

Acquisitions Editor: Tom Heine; **Developmental Editor:** Cynthia McEntire; **Assistant Editor:** Elizabeth Evans; **Copyeditor:** Bob Replinger; **Indexer:** Dan Connolly; **Permissions Manager:** Martha Gullo; **Graphic Designer:** Joe Buck; **Graphic Artist:** Kim McFarland; **Cover Designer:** Keith Blomberg; **Photographer (cover):** iStockphoto/ALEAIMAGE; **Photographer (interior):** Neil Bernstein; **Visual Production Assistant:** Jason Allen; **Art Manager:** Kelly Hendren; **Associate Art Manager:** Alan L. Wilborn; **Medical Illustrations:** © Human Kinetics; **Charts and Graphs:** Tammy Page; **Printer:** McNaughton & Gunn

We thank Fortanasce and Associates in Arcadia, California, for assistance in providing the location for the photo shoot for this book.

Human Kinetics books are available at special discounts for bulk purchase. Special editions or book excerpts can also be created to specification. For details, contact the Special Sales Manager at Human Kinetics.

Printed in the United States of America   10 9 8 7 6 5 4 3 2 1

The paper in this book is certified under a sustainable forestry program.

Human Kinetics
Website: www.HumanKinetics.com

United States: Human Kinetics
P.O. Box 5076
Champaign, IL 61825-5076
800-747-4457
e-mail: humank@hkusa.com

Canada: Human Kinetics
475 Devonshire Road Unit 100
Windsor, ON N8Y 2L5
800-465-7301 (in Canada only)
e-mail: info@hkcanada.com

Europe: Human Kinetics
107 Bradford Road
Stanningley
Leeds LS28 6AT, United Kingdom
+44 (0) 113 255 5665
e-mail: hk@hkeurope.com

Australia: Human Kinetics
57A Price Avenue
Lower Mitcham, South Australia 5062
08 8372 0999
e-mail: info@hkaustralia.com

New Zealand: Human Kinetics
P.O. Box 80
Torrens Park, South Australia 5062
0800 222 062
e-mail: info@hknewzealand.com

E5180

End Back & Neck Pain

Contents

Preface

*E*nd Back & Neck Pain focuses on the nature of, natural course of, and helpful remedies for the most common spinal pain problems. With an emphasis on education, diagnosis, prevention, and self-care, this book empowers you to participate actively in the healing of your spinal pain and keep it from recurring.

We do this in several ways. First, we provide the information that you need to understand your symptoms. Is it time to go to the emergency room or take out an ice pack? Second, we provide numerous recommendations for self-help, from medication choices to exercise to tips on body mechanics and ergonomic adaptations. The goal is to help you ease the suffering from ordinary and recurring spinal discomfort. Third, we teach you to evaluate your health care professional; can the person back up his or her credentials? Finally, if all remedies fail, we discuss the indications, risks, and expected benefits of spinal injections and surgery.

By the time an average patient finally sees a spine specialist, she or he has been to at least three doctors, tried five medications, and has seen other nonmedical specialists. The person has tried chiropractic treatments, physical therapy, acupuncture, and back and neck devices such as pillows and gravity machines. And the pain persists.

Written by three of the most prominent names in spine health, **End Back & Neck Pain** addresses the sharp, shooting, nagging, burning, aching, tight, stiff, and throbbing types of discomfort, whether they arise from a specific trauma or a vague, unknown origin. In this book, you will find relief from that nagging discomfort that you feel between your shoulder blades, the never-ending stiffness on the side of your neck, and the lingering leg pain that just won't go away.

This book covers the likely causes of 95 percent of nonthreatening spinal discomfort conditions and suggests ways to relieve that discomfort. In addition, it discusses the 5 percent of conditions that urgently need attention. *End Back & Neck Pain* is an essential guide for those suffering from complex conditions that compromise bowel or bladder function or appear suddenly with numbness and weakness in the arms, legs, or both. In these cases, the most prudent course of action is to obtain direct medical attention through a visit to your physician or local hospital.

The medical community has developed many ways to categorize and conceptualize the origin of spinal discomfort. Physicians, therapists, chiropractors, acupuncturists, and other caregivers focus on different aspects of discomfort and view the same discomfort in unique ways. Within our individual professions, we encounter a variety of opinions, which lead to vastly different approaches to care of the same spinal pain condition. You will need to consider a variety of options and theories when contemplating treatment or seeking a diagnosis. We know that what works for some will not work for all. In the area of spinal pain, no one remedy solves all problems. Unfortunately, many in the spine business believe in a one-size-fits-all cure. Therefore, you need to know what remedies are appropriate for your unique problem.

Even so, commonalities among conditions make managing spinal pain highly successful for most people. In this book we'll discuss how factors such as your office workstation setup (office ergonomics) or the ways in which you lift, carry, push, and pull (body mechanics) influence your discomfort. Similarly, your diet, level of fitness, smoking and sleeping habits, and stress management influence the prevalence of spinal pain. We'll discuss first aid for fast relief and provide stretches and exercises for common spinal maladies. In a completely accessible way, we'll discuss what structures are likely causing discomfort, how your body works to perceive the discomfort, and why it hurts in the first place. The chapter on medicines to treat spine disorders (chapter 10) will shake you up as you learn what works, what doesn't, and when medication makes it worse.

Along the way, we debunk some common myths associated with spinal pain. For example, many who have arthritis think that exercise is not appropriate. We show you why that is not so and what you can do about it. Some think that because they move all day at work they get enough exercise. We show you why that is not correct. Some think a big, soft, cushiony chair with armrests is appropriate for computer work, but that is not so. Some of you may fear that your discomfort is untreatable, that because injections or therapy or chiropractic care didn't help the next step is surgery. We discuss the details and show you why that may not be true.

In this book you will learn logical and simple self-care concepts that address the more common causes of spinal discomfort. When you have finished reading the book, you should be able to do the following:

- Understand the basic anatomy and function of the spine.
- Understand the origin of spinal pain and the symptoms that communicate what structures are most likely contributing to your spinal pain.
- Understand postural, adaptive shortening, and derangement syndromes.
- Recognize the psychological complications of back and neck pain.
- Be empowered to find and select the physician who will best be able to help you.
- Interpret the voices of pain.
- Know when to see a physician and recognize when the situation is urgent and when it is not.
- Understand what a competent physician should do when taking a history and doing a physical exam.
- Know what questions to ask your health care provider regarding the cause, treatment, and prevention of pain.
- Recognize when medication is needed, which are the best and safest options, and when they cause more harm than good.

- Understand what tests should be ordered and how to prepare yourself for those tests, taking fear out of the unknown.
- Perform emergency self-help interventions when sudden pain occurs.
- Describe and demonstrate how to set up a home or office workstation that minimizes the effects of repetitive motion and accumulative trauma.
- Perform appropriate stretches, exercises, and conditioning activities to treat your specific complaints.
- Understand surgical considerations and the conditions that are appropriate for surgical consideration and intervention.
- Know the questions and answers that you should expect from your surgeon and the risks, complications, and benefits of those interventions. Recognize that your surgeon should discuss which procedure is the best for you and carries the least risk.

For all who suffer from daily, episodic, and recurrent spinal discomfort, we provide a source of information to help you identify common causes, implement simple solutions, and begin straightforward self-help activities. You want to know what is wrong and how to fix it. This book will empower you to understand your pain and take steps to relieve it and prevent it from coming back. This approach makes the book unique. We hope that you find this book a positive step toward maintaining a happy and healthy lifestyle.

Acknowledgments

We would like to thank some of our colleagues who contributed to the development of this book and provided invaluable assistance in presenting this information. David Chang MD, who is a Princeton graduate and who works with Dr. Fortanasce and Dr. Watkins, collaborated with Dr. Watkins on the spinal injection chapter. Thanks also to spinal surgeon Robert Watkins Jr. MD; Lillian Chen DPT; and Michael Fortanasce DPT for their assistance.

Others who have greatly influence our opinions on diagnosis and treatment are our professors and colleagues: the late Vert Mooney, chief of the spinal pain services at Rancho Los Amigos Hospital (USC); Dr. Joseph Van Der Mueler; and Leshe Weiner, department chairs of neurology at USC.

Others who helped with research, typing, and preparation of the book: Laura Kennedy, Chris Foss, Annie Kershaw, Jessica Ruiz, the Dandacar brothers, Tammy Kempton, and Kathy Williams.

My wife Gayl for her psychological insights on pain. Friends who read and gave insights: Didi Astraw, Bob Bancroft, and Jeff Drier. My sisters Joan Donafrio and Elaine Fellows, and nephew Mark Fellows DPT.

A special thank you to our editors Tom Heine and Cynthia McEntire and the Human Kinetics team who worked so diligently on this project.

To my family, for whom I have always tried to do my very best, and to my parents, to whom I am extremely grateful for all they have provided for me. Thank you.

PART

I

Why Does It Hurt?

Understanding Back and Neck Pain

You wake up one morning and try to get out of bed, but a sharp, knifelike pain in your back makes you freeze. The warmth of the shower eases the pain a little, but periodically throughout the day you feel a dull ache. You begin to worry that you are getting old, that you have a serious condition that might need surgery, that this is the beginning of the end. You are not alone.

Spinal discomfort and pain are part of the human experience. We health care professionals, experts in back and neck pain, even experience it, too. Estimates are that 95 percent of the population will have at least one serious episode of spinal pain in their lives, and 84 percent will suffer multiple episodes. Of those, 33 percent will suffer from chronic pain, and 7 percent will be substantially limited in their ability to work.

Spinal pain is the second most common reason for a medical office visit and the most common reason for emergency room consultations in the United States, totaling 6 million visits per year. Spinal pain costs an estimated $110 billion per year, and another $40 billion is accrued in business expenses.

The incidence of spinal pain and location varies by occupation and gender. The low back area constitutes 70 percent of all cases, the neck 22 percent, and the midtorso 8 percent. Men are twice as likely as women to have repeated attacks, and they occur in 50 percent of those who do hard labor. Women in the white-collar workforce (secretaries, lawyers, and teachers, for example) more often have neck and shoulder blade pain. An estimated 50 percent of them have other difficulties as well, such as chronic headaches, carpal tunnel syndrome, and thoracic outlet syndrome. A spine specialist and a neurological assessment are needed in these cases. Otherwise, a non-neck problem may be mistakenly diagnosed. The number of people with spinal pain at any one time is about 60 million. An estimated 40 million suffer from chronic spinal pain.

BACK AND NECK ANATOMY

The spine is like a row of houses. Each house is a vertebra. There are 7 cervical (neck), 12 thoracic, 5 lumbar, 5 sacral, and 4 coccyx vertebrae (figure 1.1).

Feel the bones at the back of your neck and lower back. These bones, the spinous process, are like the steeples of houses. The spinous process comes off the roof of the spine, the lamina. A laminectomy is an operation in which the lamina is removed. The spine is not solid bone. It is mobile. Ligaments are present between the laminas at each level. The walls of each house are made of pillars, the pedicles.

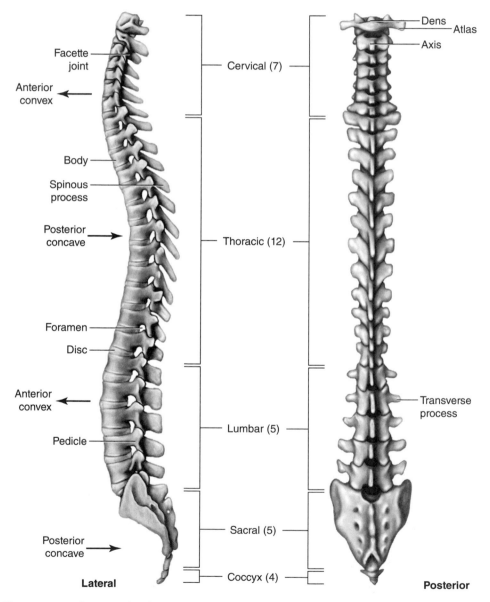

Figure 1.1   The spinal column.

The foramen is like the window of a house. The nerve exits the spinal cord through the foramen to go to the arms or legs. A foramenotomy is a surgery on the window to relieve nerve pain. The facette joints attach one vertebra to the next. Each vertebra is numbered: C1 to C7 in the neck and L1 to L5 in the lumbar region. Joints, intervertebral discs, and ligaments are located between the vertebrae. Each vertebra has some mobility because of the facette joints and ligaments. The pedicles attach to the vertebral bodies, which attach to the intervertebral discs. An intervertebral disc is a multilayered ligament that looks like a woven basket. It is laminated with multiple layers like the belts on a truck tire. The disc attaches to the vertebra above and below and allows motion between the vertebrae. Two facette joints behind the intervertebral disc make up a joint. For example, L4–L5 has a disc, two facette joints, and its own nerves. If it is injured, it hurts. The joint will swell and become inflamed like any other joint. The spinal canal runs through the vertebra. The spinal cord passes the neck, ending as the cauda equina in the low back. Ligaments under the roof and floor of the vertebra allow movement and provide structural strength and protection of the spine.

If the intervertebral disc develops a tear between its layers and its dense liquid center, or nucleous pulposa, bulges out, a disc herniation has occurred. A fragment of the disc that extrudes into the spinal canal in the neck can be extremely dangerous and may cause paralysis. A combination of the disc bulge, ligament buckling, and joint arthritis can seriously narrow the spinal canal, the living space for the spinal cord and cauda equina. The result may be a slow or sudden loss of strength, bladder control, and sensation. This condition is called spinal stenosis, a narrowing of the spinal canal.

The nerves run through the body, starting at the brain and extending all the way down to the bottom of the toes. The nerves help the doctor pinpoint the level of the spine at which the problem occurs, identify the nerve involved, and determine the specific problem, based on patient history and the physical examination.

MOVEMENTS OF THE SPINE

The spine can flex, extend, bend laterally, and twist. It is a wonderful feat of engineering. These movements change the relations of the spine anatomy. Anyone with back or neck pain knows that certain movements provoke or worsen the pain. These biomechanical functions—flexing, extending, lateral bending, and twisting—are used during the physical examination to diagnose the cause of pain. When you bend forward (flexion), the spinal canal and foramen open. When you arch your neck or back backward (extension), the spinal canal and foramen close. Patients have various symptom complexes, symptoms based on spinal motions, that take these biomechanical factors into account.

WHY DOES IT HURT?

The transmission of pain involves the exchange of chemicals within three major components of the nervous system: the peripheral nerves, spinal cord, and brain.

Origin of Anatomical Terms

Do not be intimidated by the medical anatomical terminology in this book, words such as *cauda equina*, *sciatica*, *stenosis*, *cerebrum*, *cerebellum*, and *medulla oblongata*. These terms were coined by the early fathers of anatomy. What were these great minds thinking when they came up with these tongue-twisting multisyllabic terms?

Consider the brain. The brain consists of three parts: a large part; a small, delicate, and intricate part just under the large part; and a center like a middle stalk going through the brain. The cover of the large part is yellowish, shiny, and gray, much like a candle. *Candle* in Italian is *cere*, meaning "wax." *Brum* means "big," so *cerebrum* means "big wax." The smaller delicate part, shiny and bright, is the cerebellum, from *cere* for candle and *bellum*, which means "beautiful," so cerebellum means "beautiful wax." The long middle part is the *medulla oblongata* from the Latin meaning "the long middle thing." The terms aren't so intimidating in this context.

What about the term *cauda equina*? *Cauda* means "tail," *equina* means "horse," so *cauda equina* means a "horse's tail." At the end of the spinal cord is the lumbar sacral spine. Because it gives off the nerves that become the sciatic nerve, it looks like a horse's tail.

The word *sciatic* or *sciatica* originates from the Italian word for skiing, *sciare*, which means "to cascade." The nerve cascades down from the horse's tail like a ski slope. Medical terminology is simple if you understand the language, which is Latin in this case. Pain, however, is a universal language ("Ouch!"). Each anatomical part has a particular symptom or pain, its language.

At various stages, these three components trigger, transmit, and receive electrical impulses that we perceive as unpleasant. The three types of pain-provoking stimuli are chemical (swelling), temperature (hot or cold), and direct mechanical pressure. Pain-transmitting nerve fibers have an extremely small diameter. They originate from almost every structure in the body, eventually joining with the spinal cord as it travels up to the brain.

The pain impulse instantaneously enters the thalamus, the brain's switching and sorting center. From here, the information immediately passes to three specialized areas of the brain. From the thalamus, pain impulses move to the somatosensory cortex. This area allows you to interpret physically where the discomfort comes from—your toe, lower back, or deep in your chest. This interpretation of location is important. Generally, we give more significance to symptoms that are perceived to be deeper than to those that seem more superficial. Identifying the area of discomfort is especially important when you describe your pain to your doctor or therapist. As you will learn in chapter 2, each pain-producing structure has a voice. By giving an accurate history and description of your pain, you help your doctor or therapist know which structure is talking to you.

The cerebral cortex, the active thinking part of your brain, helps decipher the urgency or severity of your symptoms and directs you to a course of action. Impulses pass to the frontal cortex as well. This area in your brain allows you to give meaning to the experience, as in "This is no good," "This really hurts," "This will go away soon," or "This needs to be addressed." This response stimulates the decision-making process so that you can decide whether to seek care. Do you miss work, skip the game, go to the hospital, or simply carry on cautiously? This decision will vary from person to person. You may already have seen your health care provider for a similar discomfort in the past and learned to be patient, confident that it will pass with a little self-help. Or you may be experiencing neck discomfort for the first time and, based on other influences such as your uncle's bad experience or a neighbor's well-intentioned advice, decide to make an urgent trip to the emergency room. The significance that we place on the spinal pain that we feel in large part dictates how we respond to it. Throughout the book, we'll provide some guidelines on what is urgent and what is not.

The pain impulse also travels to the limbic area. Here the brain assigns an emotional significance such as suffering, frustration, anxiety, or fear to the impulse. Because emotional significance is part of the pain-perception process, similar types of stimuli cause different reactions in different people. For example, the anxiety felt by someone who has never been to a dentist when he hears the drill or sees the cleaning probe may accentuate his sensation of discomfort. Or the stress and fear of losing a job or athletic ability may complicate the healing process of an otherwise manageable spine injury. Conversely, some people, such as athletes, use the emotional significance of winning to block out and endure more discomfort.

Within the brain, chemicals moderate the incoming pain signals, either dulling or amplifying the experience. These chemicals are released by the cells in the brain and are influenced by the self-help recommendations provided in later chapters. Following the guidelines that we provide will help you increase the release of pain-dulling chemicals and reduce the presence of pain-amplifying chemicals.

Emotions, fears, anxieties, and apprehensions can either open or close the valve controlling these chemicals, thereby assisting or complicating the perception of pain. Depending on a variety of factors, especially their experiences, some people have a better override mechanism than others do. This trait helps them heal and recover more quickly.

Inflammation also influences your perception of pain. In part, chronic pain arises from inflammatory processes that sensitize the nervous system, causing the nerve fibers that send pain impulses to fire more easily, frequently, or intensely. This process can occur within all centers of the pain pathway and may explain why small events can have a significant effect on those already experiencing chronic spinal pain. Modulating inflammation through exercise, diet, sleep, and relaxation, as discussed in chapter 5, is key in the overall management of chronic spinal pain.

EVALUATING YOUR PAIN

Patient attitudes have changed. In the past, patients simply said, "Fix it, doc." Now they ask, "What is my problem, and what can I do about it?" This book is about empowering you to understand why you hurt and what you can do. *End Back & Neck Pain* will be your companion. Let's begin by identifying what your spinal pain is telling you. Take the spine pain test.

Spine Pain Test

1. Is your spine pain severe, sharp, and stabbing? Yes or no.
2. Is your pain more in your arm or leg than in your spine? Yes or no.
3. Does your pain radiate from the spine down your arm or leg? Yes or no.
4. Is your pain most often associated with tingling, numbness, or burning? Yes or no.
5. Does looking up at the ceiling make your neck or arm pain worse? Yes or no.
6. Does bending, lifting, or twisting make your back pain worse? Yes or no.
7. Do you notice weakness in the painful extremity? Yes or no.
8. Does standing in one spot make the pain worse? Yes or no.
9. Do your legs get weak after walking a certain distance, such as one block? Yes or no.
10. Does rest make your pain better? Yes or no.
11. Does rest make your pain worse? Yes or no.
12. Is the pain worse in the morning? Yes or no.
13. Is your pain mainly a stiffness that gets better with exercise? Yes or no.
14. Has your pain persisted for more than three months without getting better? Yes or no.
15. Are you having difficulty doing your job because nobody appreciates how much you hurt? Yes or no.
16. Do you think that you take too much medication? Yes or no.
17. Do you sleep poorly and feel stressed most of the time? Yes or no.
18. Do you get severe calf cramps after walking a certain distance, such as one block? Yes or no.
19. Do you get up from bed and walk at night because your legs are restless? Yes or no.
20. Do you suffer from frequent cramps at night in bed? Yes or no.

For questions 1 through 10, if you answered yes five or more times, you may have nerve-related pain and should see a doctor.

If you answered yes to questions 2, 4, 7, or 9, you should see a spine specialist.

If you answered yes to questions 11, 12, or 13, you may have joint back pain and should seek therapy.

If you answered yes to questions 14, 15, 16, or 17, you may have chronic pain syndrome and should be evaluated by a pain specialist or neurologist.

If you answered yes to question 18, have your doctor check your arteries for peripheral vascular disease, which is a serious condition.

If you answered yes to question 19, you may have restless leg syndrome, which is often inherited or caused by other medications and is readily treated.

If you answered yes to question 20, you may have benign cramps because of several causes, including vitamin D mineral deficiency. Discuss with your doctor.

COMMON CAUSES OF SPINAL PAIN

Let's begin by discussing common causes of spinal pain and learning to use this information to focus treatment. This classification system is adapted from the work of Robin McKenzie, PT. We will use this classification system to outline the origin and mechanism of spinal discomfort. These causes relate equally to the cervical, thoracic, and lumbar areas.

Spinal discomfort is most common in the third to fourth decade of life and is often associated with a lack of activity at a time when people should be the most active. McKenzie observed that after college, people focus on work, career, and family demands, leading to a decline in physical fitness and an increase in a flexion-biased lifestyle. The classification system is based on these two factors: diminished fitness and a flexion-biased lifestyle.

After you identify which classification is most relevant to your spinal symptoms, you can identify the starting point of your treatment plan, whether it is an additional medical workup, a change in medication, an injection, the start of a therapy program, or home remedy activities. These three categories make explaining, understanding, and addressing spinal discomfort easier. Just as each anatomical structure has a voice, your voice in the history and observations that you make tell a story. In listening to the story, your health care team can begin to identify the proper remedy.

Many different viewpoints can come into play in categorizing spinal discomfort, depending on the person's perspective. As you consider the following, try to analyze your discomfort to discover which classification best fits your signs and symptoms. Some clinicians, depending on their viewpoint, may find fault in categorizing symptoms this way, but many of us use this format successfully. The point is not to assume that these three categories encompass all scenarios of spinal pain.

What Is a Flexion-Biased Lifestyle?

Technological progress has resulted in many of us spending a large part of our day seated. When you sit, the mid to lower cervical spine and lumbar spine tend to adopt a flexed (bent forward) position. Sitting places the disc in a position of relatively uneven loading that puts more pressure on the front aspect and less on the back. Some joints are maintained in a compressed position, whereas some muscles are routinely kept shortened. Some muscles work too hard, and others work minimally, if at all.

For many, a typical day begins with a lengthy commute to work. That activity is followed by prolonged or frequent bouts of computer and desk work, a seated lunch, and then a return to the computer in the afternoon. The workday ends with a lengthy commute home. At home, a seated dinner is followed by television and computer work throughout the evening. Weekend activities may include using the computer, watching a ball game or movie, attending an event, or relaxing to read. Missing in this lifestyle are movement and fitness activities to offset the constant and repeated spinal flexion. This constant positioning into spinal flexion—a combination of work, home, and recreational positioning—makes up the flexion-biased lifestyle that is one of two main culprits in the onset of spinal discomfort.

Nevertheless, they are an excellent starting point in identifying most spinal pain issues, and from these we can choose a logical treatment path. After you identify which category best fits your discomfort, you'll be able to use the information in chapters 3 through 7 to feel better.

The three primary classifications are postural syndrome, spinal derangement, and adaptive shortening.

Postural Syndrome

Referred to as bent finger syndrome, postural syndrome describes pain associated with a mechanical deformation of normal tissue that eventually produces discomfort. Mechanical deformation means that a prolonged strain on the tissues causes an end-of-range compression or a lengthened-position tension on a structure. Affecting the cervical, thoracic, and lumbar spine equally, spinal pain arising from a purely postural nature typically affects those in their 30s and younger. The pain is always local, never radiating, and never constant, and it is not produced with movement. The discomfort is intermittent, coming and going, often for periods at a time. Associated with a sedentary job, a lack of exercise, or constant unchanging positions, postural syndrome symptoms arise as the person actively moves into the faulty position, often unaware that she or he is doing so. The person often is not even aware that the positioning is the cause of the symptoms.

To illustrate postural syndrome, bend your index finger back until it begins to hurt. Notice where it hurts and what happens to the discomfort when you release the finger. The discomfort was local to the finger joint (nonradiating), occurred over time when a prolonged tension was applied in an end-range position (mechanical deformation in an end-of-range motion position), and eased when the pressure was released (intermittent discomfort). This discomfort fits the definition of postural syndrome pain because it comes and goes as the finger moves into and out of the position of pain elicited by the mechanical deformation of your pushing on it.

Now bend your index finger back again, but this time resist the force with some muscular effort at the finger. As one hand pushes on the finger, use the finger muscles to oppose the pressure, maintaining the finger in a neutral, at-rest position. Do you feel discomfort? Does the joint feel compressed, jammed, or tense? Likely not. The joint and surrounding tissues are happily in the middle of their available positions, far from tension or compression forces that cause the nerve fibers to signal pain. By using muscular effort to oppose the symptom-producing forces, you have found the key to the treatment of your spinal problem.

Postural syndrome is found in school-aged children, often girls, who stand with their knees hyperextended (locked fully straight). This stance creates irritation and pain of the tissues around the knee, often extending to the lower back, and mid-thoracic and cervical spine. Add the weight of a backpack, and the spine becomes highly susceptible to discomfort.

Slumping in a chair for hours while reading or using a computer leaves adults susceptible to postural-related pain in the midthoracic area. The paraspinals—long,

---

Is It Postural Syndrome?

To know whether a postural syndrome treatment approach is right for you, ask yourself these questions:

- Do you spend hours at a time on the same task in the same position every day?
- Do you have a sedentary job? A sedentary lifestyle?
- Are you 30 years old or younger?
- Does the discomfort come and go and vary in intensity and frequency? Does it get better after you change positions or exercise?
- Is the discomfort confined to the back? Is it annoying or gnawing but not urgent or intense? Is it nonradiating (that is, the pain doesn't move down the arm or leg)?

---

thin muscles that span many spinal segments from the neck to the tailbone—gradually succumb to the force of gravity and lose their ability to hold you upright, especially after several hours in the poor position. As you slouch, those muscles are stretched (a mechanical deformation) and, along with other spinal structures, gradually lead to the perception of discomfort. As the overstretched muscles tire, knots develop, creating that low-grade, dull, gnawing ache, perhaps between the shoulder blades or across the neck. Ropey bands within the muscle contribute to chemical irritation of the nerve endings by diminishing blood flow and local oxygen transport. The reaction of these bands and the symptoms that follow are the secondary results caused by postural syndrome. They are what cause you grief.

Other scenarios that may result in postural syndrome include holding the phone against your shoulder and ear; driving a delivery truck or commuting a long way; prolonged standing to cook, clean, or shop; typing or reading; or performing desk-related job activities. In each case, the spinal pain sufferer can move into and fully out of the symptom-provoking position but in most cases does not because he or she is not even aware that the position is causing the discomfort in the first place.

Common spinal diagnoses associated with postural syndrome include cervical, thoracic, or lumbar strain; mechanical low back pain; headaches; and muscle strain. Given the mechanism of the symptoms, the treatment for postural syndrome clearly is exercise, specifically exercises designed to strengthen the muscles needed to hold you in the proper, non-symptom-producing position—not that biking, jogging, and softball won't help.

For those with discomfort in the cervical area, postural syndrome commonly involves the muscles of the midback and shoulder blades (figure 1.2) and the short neck flexors along the front of the neck. For those with lower back symptoms, strengthening the lower abdominals, gluteal (buttock) muscles, and lateral hip muscles is of primary importance. Just as supporting your finger as you pushed it

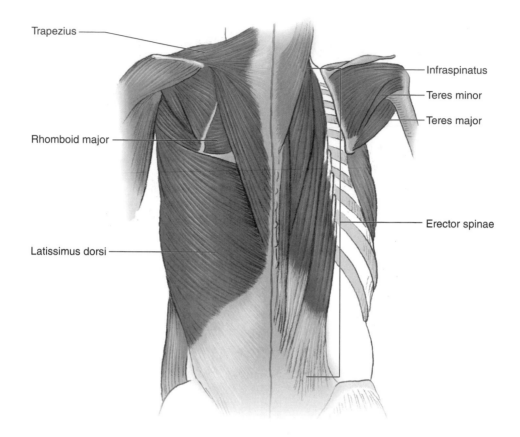

Trapezius

Infraspinatus

Teres minor

Teres major

Rhomboid major

Erector spinae

Latissimus dorsi

Figure 1.2   Muscles of the back.

back eliminated discomfort, the treatment for postural syndrome pain should be to strengthen the muscles that support the spine and learn to correct the faulty positions that are causing the discomfort. For specific exercises, see chapter 4.

To help recognize the irritating factor, pay attention to your positioning during the day and try to correlate it to the onset of your discomfort. After you identify the likely cause, you can try to change that position and start strengthening activities to offset the position.

Spinal Derangement

What McKenzie called derangement syndrome does not refer literally to your state of mind, although the discomfort may make you figuratively crazy. Instead, the term refers to a condition of the spinal disc. Spinal disc bulges, herniations, and annular tears are common conditions that affect the spinal discs. Generally, about one-third of disc problems occur in the cervical spine, about two-thirds in the lumbar spine, and a small percentage (roughly 2 percent) in the thoracic area. More prevalent in males than females, disc dysfunction is most common in the 25- to 50-year-old age group and is associated with a flexion-biased lifestyle. Onset of most discogenic conditions is usually nontraumatic, occurring gradually over time instead of resulting from a one-time traumatic event such as a fall or car accident. Although the precipitating event may have been writing a lengthy report, working in the yard over the weekend, lifting a baby from the crib, or bending repeatedly while sorting files at work, the origin of the problem likely had been brewing for many months, even years.

Discogenic-related symptoms follow a classic presentation. Their voice is clear and seldom garbled. Symptoms of discogenic origin are episodic, recurring over time, each episode a little more severe and longer lasting than the prior one. Typically, symptoms begin with mild stiffness and ache and resolve quickly and without lasting deficit. As each episode passes, the discomfort becomes more debilitating until treatment is sought.

Symptoms in the cervical area often include painful stiffness when turning the head. Discomfort may or may not radiate into the arm. A deep, fist-size ache between the shoulder blades, known as a Cloward's sign, is a common complaint. Often, looking down and turning the head are limited. Jolting or jarring activities such as driving on a bumpy road are painful.

When pain is in the lumbar area, sitting and bending worsen the discomfort but walking generally eases the pain. Lying on the side or back with the feet up also often helps ease pain because these positions generate the lowest intradiscal pressure.

Attention, Weekend Warriors

Raphael is in his early 50s. While playing tennis one weekend, Raphael tweaked his lower back. He felt no specific pop or pull but a gradually increasing sensation of stiffness in his lower back during the match. Within a short time, he could not continue. Several hours later, he could barely move.

Raphael had felt this before, but this episode was the worst that he had experienced. He felt discomfort in the left side of his lower back and into his buttocks. He felt no leg pain, numbness, or tingling. His pain was worse in the mornings. Sitting, moving from sitting to standing, and bending to put on his shoes were difficult to do. He had trouble bending to brush his teeth, wash dishes, or pick up even light items. After he was upright, Raphael could walk without pain. He also felt fine when he lay on his back with his feet up or on his side. He was able to prop himself up on his elbows and do a series of repeated back bends, which he used as the starting point for his self-help program.

Does this sound familiar to you weekend warriors? Raphael's history is classic: recurrent episodes of discomfort, each one worse than the previous; inability to maneuver into forward-flexion activities that increase disc pressure; unilateral discomfort not typically past the knee; pain worse in the morning yet better in the middle of the day; and pain improvement with walking or lying on the side. Raphael's classic presentation of symptoms led to a diagnosis of facette joint arthritis and an easily identifiable treatment approach: ice over the lower back, instruction in proper body mechanics to minimize flexion forces during activity, and back-bending maneuvers. Within 2 days Raphael was well on his way toward feeling better. About 10 days later he felt almost right again.

Forward bending produces symptoms and is often the most difficult movement to do. Coughing and sneezing are often painful, and discomfort increases when moving from sitting to standing. Usually, symptoms are worse in the morning, ease as the day progresses, and flare up again by the end of the day.

In all cases, symptoms may be in the center of the spine (central) or off to one side (unilateral), or they may radiate to the arm or leg (peripheral or referred). Generally, if the discomfort moves away from the spine or farther down the arm or leg, the condition is considered to have worsened. If the symptoms move more centrally toward the spine, it is considered a sign of healing. In fact, you may experience a more severe and noticeable pain closer to the spine as the symptoms in your arm or leg abate. This centralization of symptoms, although more uncomfortable in one spot, is a positive part of the healing process.

For those with derangement syndrome, activities that increase flexion pressure tend to worsen symptoms, and activities that lessen flexion pressure tend to ease symptoms. Lying on your side lessens disc pressure and generally feels good. Sitting, bending, and leaning over increase disc pressure and generally are not easily tolerated.

To understand the mechanism of discogenic pathology, visualize a jelly donut, which has many characteristics similar to those of a spinal disc. In both items, a viscous, gel-like center is surrounded by a firm but moveable outer layer. If you grab a donut and press evenly on the top and bottom, the donut will not deform much. If you push down on the front part of the donut, the jelly in the center likely will be forced to the back of the donut, away from the pressure. If the donut has a small hole or crack, the jelly may eventually squeeze out through the crack, possibly spilling out along the side. Jelly that simply presses against the outer edges of the donut would be analogous to what your doctor refers to as a disc bulge. Jelly that actually oozes out from the donut would be similar to what your doctor would call a disc herniation.

The point is that the central nucleus responds to asymmetrical pressure placed on the disc. As you bend forward, pressure is placed on the nucleus toward the back. As you bend backward, pressure is placed on the nucleus in a more forward direction. The posterior structures are the most innervated with pain fibers. Therefore, with repeated and prolonged bending, pressure on the disc continually forces the nucleus toward the posterior. As fissures develop within the annular bands, the center material migrates toward the back of the disc where the more pain sensitive structures are located. These include the posterior longitudinal ligament, spinal nerve roots, and spinal cord. As the disc material moves out, the disc height may gradually decrease, setting up conditions such as spinal stenosis, degenerative disc disease, and joint arthropathy. These conditions are secondary to disc derangement and occur later in life, generally in the early 50s or later.

An MRI result that shows a disc bulge implies that the annular wall is intact, which is a good thing because the hydrostatic mechanism (pressure gradient) within the disc is intact. Much like a water balloon, it may change its shape when it is pressed on, but the water does not spill out. The disc often responds to treatments such as training in proper body mechanics to minimize flexion pressures and performing repeated movements that use back bending to offset the flexion pressure. Positions and movements of the spinal column influence the position of the nucleus either adversely or as a therapeutic intervention.

An MRI that indicates a herniation or rupture implies that the disc wall has been breached and that the center material is extruding. The hydrostatic mechanism is no longer intact. Interventions that work on the concept of pressure are not as effective. Fortunately, other treatment options are effective, such as exercises, stretching, and localized ice to address inflammation.

Is It Derangement Syndrome?

To know whether a derangement syndrome treatment approach is right for you, ask yourself these questions:

- Are you 25 to 50 years old?
- Do you spend most of your week sitting or bending forward?
- Is the discomfort episodic, each time stronger, more limiting, and longer lasting than the prior bout?
- Do you feel better as the day progresses but worse in the morning and by the end of the day?
- Does extending the neck or lower back feel good but looking down or bending forward hurt?
- Does it hurt more when you cough or sneeze? When you move from sitting to standing? When you bend to brush your teeth, wash your face, slip on your socks and shoes, or get into your car?

Symptoms of a discogenic origin generally elicit a yes response to most of these questions.

Adaptive Shortening

Unlike postural syndrome, adaptive shortening implies an inability to move actively out of a pain-producing position. Over time, the connective tissue and muscles become shortened and tight, the result of prolonged, repeated positioning in one posture without adequate stretching out of that posture. The key characteristic in this group is a functional loss of motion—an inability to move into a more comfortable position because a shortness of some tissue is preventing that from happening. You're not aware of it, of course, because the body does a good job of finding alternative motions to accomplish what you want it to do. Regardless, the shortness of some tissues creates imbalances that cause pain over time.

Affecting the cervical, thoracic, and lumbar spine equally, spinal pain arising from adaptive shortening typically occurs to those in their 30s and older. The condition is most prevalent in those over 50 years old. People with a generally sedentary lifestyle and those who tend to maintain the same position for most of the day are susceptible, especially as they age. Symptoms may be local or radiating, sometimes intense, and may seem urgent, especially with diagnoses of radiculopathy or sciatica. Symptoms usually are not constant and ease with a change of position. Complaints may be described as annoying, and functional limitations are present, especially when walking or looking or reaching up. These patients tend to present with diagnoses of spinal stenosis, cervical or lumbar radiculopathy, sciatica, degenerative joint disease, or neck or low back pain. The stiffening of the tissues with age and the shortening of the tissues attributed to a flexion-biased lifestyle often are the roots of the problem.

A normal lifestyle can feature an abundance of one type of activity, such as sitting, at the expense of another, such as exercise. For example, consider an accountant, secretary, truck driver, and airline pilot. Each has a job that requires a lot of sitting. If constant sitting is unopposed by stretching, over time the hip flexors in the front of the hips, calves, lower back connective tissues, upper chest, suboccipitals at the base of the skull, and some of the front neck muscles shorten. The head tends to jut forward, and the shoulder blades round toward the front. The midback rounds as well, and the lower back becomes excessively lordotic (bent back). The tight lower leg muscles limit hip and ankle motion so that when walking the pelvic girdle tilts forward and the spine moves into an excessively lordotic position. Especially during walking, the shortness of muscle length leads to added shear and torsion stresses through the spine that lead to degenerative joint disease over time.

Consider a postal carrier, airline mechanic, warehouse supervisor, and car salesman. Each has a job that entails a lot of standing or walking. If this standing and walking is repeated and unopposed by stretching, over time such people will develop movement limitations similar to those who sit all the time, only in the opposite direction. This is the process by which adaptive shortening occurs.

Without offsetting the constant or excessive positions assumed during the week, the body adapts to a new normal and shortens to fit that position. Discomfort is the result when people attempt activities that place tension on those shortened structures when they move out of the usual position. For those who sit, activities involving standing, walking, shopping, cooking, cleaning, and recreation such as golf or tennis—activities that require extension—tend to produce symptoms. For those who stand and walk all week, activities that require bending such as gardening, reading, painting, or computer use seem to elicit symptoms. As the adaptively shortened tissues are stretched, discomfort is felt.

For those with postural syndrome, strengthening is paramount; for those with adaptive shortening, stretching is the remedy. By elongating the shortened tissues, you relieve the cause of the symptoms. As a result, you can use movement patterns that are more natural, use movement options that are more normal, and engage in more day-to-day activities without discomfort.

Those in this category of spinal pain are older than those in the postural group. Connective tissue is made up in part of proteins, of which elastin is a component. The elastin gives the tissue a springy nature, allowing it to elongate or return to its resting shape as necessary. Elastin gives your skin the bounce back characteristic that you see when you pull or push on it. As we age, elastin is gradually replaced with a thicker, more fibrous tissue that is less malleable and less giving with movement.

This new tissue doesn't stretch as easily. When it is repeatedly placed in shortened positions such as when you sit all day or stand and reach to the right all day, the tissue tends to conform more readily to those positions. Repeated positioning in conjunction with tissues that become less elastic and more fibrous as we age sets the groundwork for adaptive shortening. Through this process adaptive shortness is created.

Is It Adaptive Shortening Syndrome?

To know whether an adaptive shortening treatment approach is right for you, ask yourself these questions:

- Do you spend hours at a time on the same task in the same position each day?
- Do you have a sedentary job? A sedentary lifestyle?
- Are you 50 years old or older? Adaptive shortening is more common in those over 50, although it can show up in those 30 and older.
- Does the pain vary in intensity? Does it feel better in certain positions but worse when you change positions?
- Does looking down or turning your head cause pain in your neck? Are your shoulder blades rounded forward and your upper back curved (hunched) forward?
- Is your spine often overly extended (bent back) during long parts of your day?
- When you walk, do you notice that your pelvic girdle rotates (twists) more than the spines of others?
- When you bend forward to touch the floor, is your range of motion less when your knees are locked straight and more when your knees are slightly bent?
- Is the pain localized to your back or neck, or does it radiate into the arm or leg?
- Does stretching ease the pain but engaging in activities such as sports or work aggravate your symptoms?

Watch others walk and then assess your own gait. If you have adaptive shortening, you may notice that your pelvic girdle seems to rotate more than others'. This occurs because the front of your hips and back of your lower legs are likely very tight. When you lack motion in one plane, the body compensates by adding movement in another plane. As you attempt to move in a forward direction, the tightness creates a movement torque into rotation of the pelvic girdle and lower back, thereby causing torsion forces discussed in chapter 6. These forces lead to many of the symptoms discussed throughout the book.

If you have adaptive shortening, your ability to bend forward and touch the floor will be less with your knees locked straight and better when they are slightly bent. In either case, you should notice that your spine doesn't seem to move much. Most of the motion comes by hinging through your hips or upper back, not your lower back.

By analyzing your common postures and positions during the day, you can begin to identify what may be staying shortened, thereby understanding what needs to be stretched. The stretches covered in chapter 4 often go a long way in mitigating discomfort. The key is to stay consistent with stretching because often the dynamics of your day will not change significantly. The advantage of a program that relies on stretching for improvement is that stretching is easy to do. It doesn't require a special trip to the gym, and it can be done in several small bouts during the day, often while you are doing something else. You don't need to find 15 or 20 minutes a day to exercise. For example, you can easily stretch the backs of your lower legs while standing and talking to a friend on the phone or stretch the front of your chest on a door frame as you wait for the water to boil or the microwave to chime.

TAKE ACTION

If you are looking for some quick help, you may want to jump to chapter 3, which covers immediate first aid. The following chapters on self-help, exercise, and body mechanics will show you what to do for issues related to postural syndrome, derangement syndrome, and adaptive shortening. Keep reading. Now that you know how pain is transmitted, interpreted, and modulated and you understand some of the basic factors that lead to the onset of spinal discomfort, let's look at basic anatomy and the voices of pain. This topic will help to explain how and why the interventions offered later in the book may be effective.

Listening to the Voices of Pain

To a neurologist, orthopedist, or other pain doctor, the anatomy of pain means understanding what part of the spine has been injured and what the pain tells us. You need to listen to what the pain is telling you because each anatomical structure has its own voice. Symptoms such as tingling, weakness, and urinary problems also contribute to the voice of pain.

Anyone who has had severe acute spine pain will tell you that spine pain is like many voices all screaming at once. How do you distinguish each voice of pain? Spine pain is like a symphony. A trained ear can pick out each instrument—the horns from the strings from the piano—because it is aware of the distinctive sounds of each instrument. In the case of pain, each anatomical part has a distinctive localization, quality, radiation, and associated symptoms such as weakness, numbness, or bowel or bladder incontinence. Each speaks its own language. The anatomy of pain is what your doctor uses to build a case or, in medical terms, a diagnosis of the cause or origin for your pain. An effective treatment plan is built on the proper diagnosis.

The lumbosacral (L-S) and cervical spine (C-S) have the same anatomical parts, except the lumbosacral spine has the cauda equina and the cervical spine has the spinal cord. Figure 2.1 shows the three types of vertebrae: cervical, thoracic, and lumbar. The neck (cervical) and back (thoracic and lumbar) spines are different in that they have different shapes. The neck bones are smaller and rounder so that you can easily bend and turn your neck. The low back bones are larger and squarer so that they can bear all your weight.

Each anatomical part has a particular symptom or pain, its language (see table 2.1). Listen to what your pain is telling you.

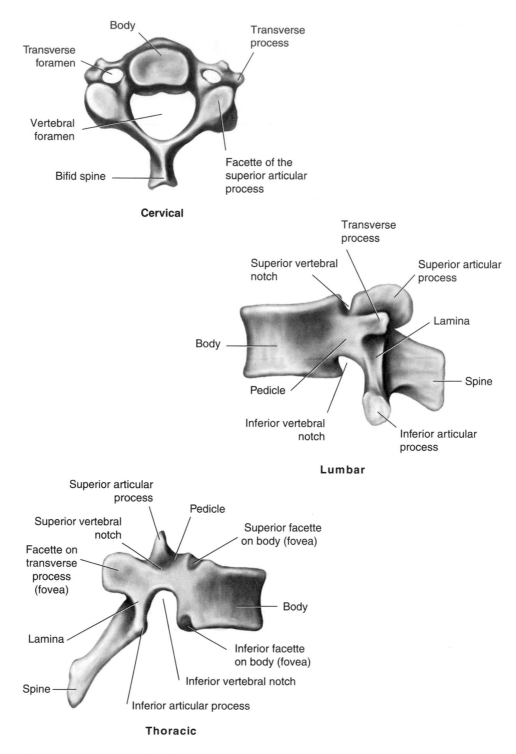

Figure 2.1 Cervical, lumbar, and thoracic vertebrae.

Table 2.1 Common Types of Back and Neck Pain

	Onset	Quality and severity of pain (intensity scale of 1 to 10)	Location of pain	Radiation of pain	Actions that provoke or worsen pain	Actions that ease pain	Associated symptoms
Nerve radicular pain (page 22)	Often sudden	Stabbing, electric shock, deep aching, worst pain ever felt Can be a 10 on a scale of 1 to 10	Localized neck or low back pain often felt below the shoulder or the buttocks in a narrow band-like distribution Extremity pain can be more severe than spine pain	Along nerve path (down the arm or leg, for example); often associated with tingling along a specific, well-defined path	Worsened by lifting or twisting; extension of neck or back; exercise or activity during flare up	Eased by resting or lying on one's side with legs bent Ice application and anti-inflammatory medication ease pain	Often feels like pins and needles in a nerve root pattern; less often causes weakness in a nerve root pattern In severe case, causes bowel and bladder problems May cause severe neck or very severe back pain
Joint or facet pain (page 25)	Often gradual over several months though can be sudden	Deep to dull aching, occasionally a sharp catch in the neck or back, stiffness after waking or after sitting for a long time At first, 5 to 8 on a scale of 1 to 10, then generally 2 to 4	Always localized in the neck or low back 90 to 100 percent back pain	May radiate to the trapezius or shoulders In the low back, may radiate to the buttocks Does not radiate below shoulder or buttock	Worsened by extension of neck or back or twisting; forward bending also may be troublesome Pain comes on when resting after activity	Eased by movement and exercise, especially stretching	Usually none
Spinal stenosis (page 30)	Slow over months or years	Dull ache to severe deep ache in neck or back After standing or walking, tingling in legs (pseudoclaudication), heavy feeling, or weakness; clumsiness in arms Generally 2 to 5 at first but worsens to 9 or 10 on a scale of 1 to 10	Located in neck or back Percent of pain in spine or neck versus arm or leg varies depending on cause Extremity pain worsens with progression	Often radiates bilaterally down arms or legs	Worsened by extension of neck or back as if looking up, standing, walking	Eased by bending forward, sitting, or riding a stationary bicycle	Bilateral arm or leg numbness and weakness Bowel and bladder problems because of genital and anal numbness
Muscle tear or pull (page 27)	Sudden after injury	Localized sharp or deep ache At first, very severe, 6 to 8 on a scale of 1 to 10, then eases to 3 to 5	Localized over muscle injured 100 percent spinal muscle, 0 percent extremity	Pain stays in injured area	Worsened by use of the injured muscle or movement that requires muscle contraction	Eased by ice application and resting of affected muscle	Weakness, swelling, or bruising without sensory loss in muscle injured
Disc pain (page 27)	Usually gradual although may occur suddenly	Dull ache Rating of 2 to 5 on a scale of 1 to 10	Spine or extremity	May stay local to spine or radiate into arm or leg	Worsened by bending, lifting, twisting, or looking down	Eased by rest and extension activities	None but often progresses to joint or nerve symptoms

(continued)

Table 2.1   *continued*

	Onset	Quality and severity of pain (intensity scale of 1 to 10)	Location of pain	Radiation of pain	Actions that provoke or worsen pain	Actions that ease pain	Associated symptoms
Spinal cord injury (page 30)	Sudden or gradual	Varies by cause (spinal stenosis, fracture, herniated disc) May have no pain at first	Varies as to cause (fracture, spinal stenosis)	Mixed	Worsened with flexion (bending forward) or extension (bending backward)	Eased by rest	Paralysis or sensory loss below level of injury and bladder and bowel symptoms with time
Ligament pain (page 30)	Gradual	Dull ache Rating of 2 to 4 on a scale of 1 to 10	Localized over injury at first 100 percent spine	No radiation	Worsened with movement or end range position that creates tension in ligament	Varies	Often associated with joint symptoms
Bone pain (page 31)	Sudden	Piercing Rating of 8 or 9 on a scale of 1 to 10	Very localized over spinous process 100 percent spine	Pain stays over area but often causes muscle spasm	Worsened by lying down Bending or twisting provokes severe pain	Varies	Can cause symptoms of nerve pain of the spinal cord or nerve root History of osteopenia or trauma in women
Psychological pain (page 32)	Varies; may be sudden or gradual	Pain with feelings of dread or impending doom; anxious feeling that is worse at night; aching Physiological pain may be intensified 10-fold by anxiety; not uncommon for pain to be rated a constant 10 Occasionally experience tingling hands and feet with shortness of breath	Diffuse over entire neck or back, depending on origin of pain	Radiation variable and at times described as "all over"	Stress, work, relationships, marriage, financial problems Worse when standing, walking, or sitting	Improves with sleep and administration of an antidepressant	Anxiety, insomnia, early waking, dread, thoughts of suicide

NERVE RADICULAR PAIN

Nerves (figure 2.2) have the most intricate anatomy and the most distinctive voices and symptoms. You must appreciate nerve pain because this voice signifies danger that may be permanent and lead to disability or paralysis. A study done of 100 patients with acute severe low back pain of a nerve origin showed that 90 percent were able to describe distinctly that the pain felt was nerve pain—not joint, muscle, or disc—although some of these structures may have also been involved.

Nerve pain has several elements—quality, quantity, location, radiation, and associated symptoms—which include dermatomal (sensation) and myotomal (muscle) and end organs if the affected nerve supplies the bowel and bladder. Let's listen to the nerves, one of the most important parts of the spine.

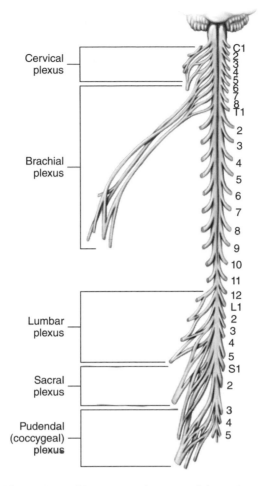

Cervical
plexus

Brachial
plexus

Lumbar
plexus

Sacral
plexus

Pudendal
(coccygeal)
plexus

C1
2
3
4
5
6
7
8
T1
2
3
4
5
6
7
8
9
10
11
12
L1
2
3
4
5
S1
2
3
4
5

Figure 2.2 Nerves coming out of the spine.

Quality, Quantity, Location, and Radiation

When irritated or crushed, a nerve produces a stabbing, knifelike pain of horrible proportions. Patients describe it as the worst pain that they ever felt, like a knife in the back or neck, or a toothache. It also may feel like an electric shock. Nerve pain is loud and always severe. On a scale of 1 to 10, with 1 being little pain and 10 being excruciating pain, nerve pain often rates a 5 to 10.

Nerve pain has a distinctive location and radiation. A nerve is like a telephone line with connections. For example, pain in the hand may originate 3 feet (90 cm) away in the neck. Therefore, the pain can begin in the neck and radiate down the arm all the way to the hand. Neck pain that radiates below the shoulder to the hand or low back pain that radiates below the knee to the foot often is from a nerve root, where the nerve exits the foramen, or window.

A characteristic of nerve pain is that it more often is in the extremity, the arm or leg, than in the neck or low back. In several studies in which patients were asked to distribute their pain, extremity verses spine, patients with definite nerve pain localized the pain to be greater in the extremity than in the spine; for example, they attributed 70 percent of the pain to the extremity versus 30 percent to the back. A distinct difference is found between nerve pain and pain from other structures such as the bone, muscle, or disk, in which pain is usually localized completely in the spine or radiates only in the neck to the shoulder or in the low back to the buttocks.

Modifiers of Nerve Pain

An important sign of nerve pain is what makes symptoms worse and what improves them. Identifying what provokes the pain is important. Nerve pain may be provoked if you do a straight leg raise (see page 155). Nerve pain is worsened by movement, especially bending, twisting, and lifting. Typically, pain improves with rest, especially when you lie on your back or on your side with your legs flexed. Pain that originates from other structures such as the facette joint may be made worse with rest and improve with movement.

Nerve Pain's Unique Voice

The dermatome and myotome of nerve pain resemble the names of musical instruments. (Dermatome refers to the sensory distribution of a nerve. Myotome refers to the motor or strength distribution of a nerve.) On a string instrument, each string gives a distinctive resonance that tells a trained musician what note it is. The myotome and dermatome of nerve pain tells a well-trained doctor exactly what nerve is causing the problem.

When injured, the sensory fibers produce a tingling sensation like pins and needles or sometimes a burning sensation. These are the most common sensory symptoms and must not be confused with pain. Pain is an unpleasant feeling that is sharp, aching, or throbbing. Pain can arise from most of the spinal structures, so pain in itself does not mean that a nerve is injured. Pain with tingling, however, does. If the nerve is completely severed, you will have no feeling.

A trained musician listening to a symphony can distinguish the strings from the horns and the piano forte from the percussion instruments. When evaluating nerve pain, trained physicians distinguish the quality of the pain, its radiation, the things that provoke or improve it, and the things that worsen or aggravate the pain. The distinctive elements associated only with nerve injury are specific sensory, motor, and bowel and bladder signs.

For example, an injured S1 nerve (S for sciatic, 1 for the first level) causes pain down the back of the leg to the lateral part of the knee and then to the ankle and the foot, especially the lateral part of the foot near the fifth toe. An injury to the L5 nerve root causes tingling and sensory changes to the large toe. Each nerve has its own voice. Luckily, this voice is the same in every person, making the diagnostic process easier. Your doctor should be able to tell you what nerve is involved based on his or her evaluation of your pain. The correct diagnostic test (EMG or MRI scan) and physical exam will confirm the diagnosis.

The myotome refers to the muscles to which a particular nerve goes. The myotome distribution for the S1 nerve is the gastrocnemius, or calf, muscle that allows you to

> ⚠ Beware. When a nerve is involved, it is a medical emergency. If your doctor cannot see you, consider going to the emergency room, especially if you have bowel and bladder symptoms or progressive weakness. Don't wait!

stand on your toes and is important for running. An L3 or L4 myotome goes to the quadriceps, or thigh, muscle. Just as a pianist can tell the key played by its tone, a trained physician can tell the exact nerve involved by its distinctive myotomal and dermatomal voices.

If the entire bundle of spinal nerve roots (cauda equina) is injured, the nerves to the bowel and bladder are impaired. You will have difficulty controlling urination or bowel function. You may also experience numbness to the saddle area around your rectum and genitals. This important voice should never be ignored.

JOINT OR FACETTE PAIN

The facette is a joint. A facette is round and looks like a face, hence the word *facette*, which is from *face* and *ette*, or little. The facette joint has a superior (above) part and an inferior (below) part that include facettes from adjacent vertebrae (figure 2.3). It has a covering, or membrane, that has many small blood vessels and fluid in between so that the joint flows smoothly and allows the bending, twisting, and extending movements that are vital to swinging a golf club, bending forward to brush your teeth, or extending to put that light bulb in the ceiling fixture.

The facette is also well innervated, meaning that it has sensation nerves going to it that connect it to other parts of the spine, usually one level above the affected area and two levels below it. The facettes have input for multiple spinal levels.

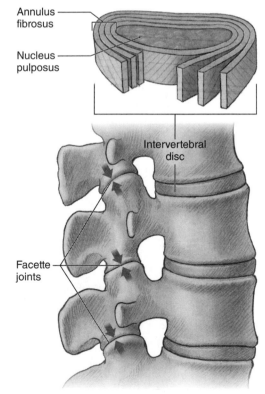

Quality, Quantity, Location, and Radiation

The pain can be acute or stabbing, but more often it is described as a dull ache or stiffness. Facette pain radiates differently than nerve pain. Facette back pain never goes below the knee and rarely goes below the buttocks. Facette neck pain never goes below the trapezius or shoulder. Facette pain usually is given a 2 to 4 on a scale of 1 to 10, but in acute cases it can get an 8.

Figure 2.3 Structure of the vertebrae.

Aggravating factors for facette pain in the low back and neck are activities such as lying down or sitting for 15 minutes or more. Often facette pain is worse in the morning. Usually this is a stiff, aching pain that improves with moving and stretching, which is different from nerve pain. Back extension, or bending backward, may worsen pain. Bending backward pushes the facettes together, irritating the joint.

The facette is often injured while playing golf or participating in other twisting activities. The pain is not necessarily noted when the golfer is swinging, but minutes or even hours later. The same is true if the injury occurs while you are working at your desk, gardening, or housecleaning. You may feel fine while doing it, but your back aches a half hour later. The pain can come on suddenly, such as when brushing your teeth.

Often facette pain is called the pain of long-earned wear and tear. For the secretary, it is the constant bending over to pull files; for the electrician or dentist, it is the twisting of the neck to fix what the job requires. This is the pain of the shortening adaptive syndrome.

Facette Degeneration

Over time, normal wear and tear and bleeding into the facette joint cause inflammation or the formation of bone spurs that jut out into the foramen where the nerve lives. In time, these bone spurs can stab into the nerve, causing tingling and loss of strength. This bony arthritis is an inflammation in the joint. (*Arthro* means "joint.") This inflammation also can narrow the central canal of the lumbosacral or cervical spine. When this occurs, you are in big trouble. (See the section on spinal stenosis on page 30, later in this chapter.) In a way, this inflammation is the body attacking itself with substances such as tumor necrosis factor (TNF). The effect of these substances can be stopped by the use of anti-inflammatory drugs such as aspirin, ibuprofen, and others. Anti-inflammatory drugs relieve facette pain. Facette degeneration often precedes nerve pain, but not always.

Take an anti-inflammatory drug before any activity that will aggravate the joint. For example, take an ibuprofen or naprosyn one hour before you play golf. Taking the medication after performing the activity is not as effective.

MUSCLE, LIGAMENT, AND TENDON PAIN

Injuries to the muscles, ligaments, or tendons are categorized as soft-tissue injuries. A muscle injury might be the most painful, but injuries to the ligaments and tendons are the most enduring and limiting. Fortunately, ligament and tendon injuries are rare. Muscle injury is more common and is frequently seen in weekend warriors who play softball, tennis, golf, basketball, or other recreational sports.

Muscles have many blood vessels. Muscles are innervated by nerves from the spine in a distinct myotome fingerprint. Because the muscles of the upper chest, upper back, shoulder, and pelvis, including the buttocks and thighs, are of great size and strength, they provide stability and ease of movement to the neck and low back. When injured, these muscles spasm, limiting motion to prevent further pain. In any injury—bone, nerve, facette, or tendon—the nervous system causes the muscle to spasm to protect the whole spinal circuitry, sort of like a short circuit switch. The muscle spasm inactivates the spine and shuts it down. When a muscle goes into spasm, the blood supply to that muscle is cut off, further injuring the muscle.

A violent action can cause the muscle to tear. But even when the muscle is not torn, a reflex spasm to protect the joint will cause it to shut down. The muscle spasm contracts the muscle, making it reduce its size by half at times, and squeezes on the blood supply. The muscle is unable to get proper nutrition and oxygen, which injures the muscle and inhibits the removal of toxins. The muscle breaks down and becomes inflamed, creating additional problems. This is collateral damage. The muscle is involuntarily in spasm, and the body will begin to attack itself with cytokines. Cytokines are the artilleries that the body uses to defend itself. They destroy any tissue that they are released on, even normal muscle. In most injuries to the nerves, facettes, or bones of the spine, collateral damage to the muscle will occur.

The quality of muscle pain may be sharp at first and then become a deep soreness localized over the area of injury. If you try to use that muscle, you will feel the tenderness and pain. When a doctor palpates the muscle, he or she can feel the knot. That knot is the swelling caused by the inflammation and sometimes by blood or other fluid seeping into the injured area.

In the acute stage of injury or spasm, ice helps and heat makes it worse. Heat draws more blood and causes increased collateral damage to the area. Ice slows down the whole inflammatory process. Remember, facettes and soft tissues do not have the same fingerprint as nerves do. Injuries to facettes and soft tissues do not create sensory loss or weakness in a distinctive dermatomal or myotomal pattern. Here the weakness from soft-tissue injury is limited to the muscle or tendon involved.

A health care professional must be knowledgeable in neuroanatomy. Unfortunately, many are not so trained. Each nerve goes to a particular muscle. The well-trained spine specialist can identify the origin of the injury.

Movement makes muscle pain worse, but the pain is localized over the injured muscle. (Remember that movement causes nerve pain to radiate down the arm or leg and is often associated with sensory or motor changes.) Rest helps a torn muscle, as does ice at first and anti-inflammatory drugs.

DISC PAIN

The vertebral disc (figure 2.4) consists of two parts. The annulus fibrocartilaginous, which is made of dense fibers and cartilage, surrounds a soft yet dense liquidlike mass called the nucleus pulposus (NP). The NP acts as a cushion or shock absorber to the spine so that when you land on your rear end you don't fracture your spine. The NP takes the thrust and torque and changes shape, giving elasticity to the spinal column.

Think of the annulus fibrosa (AF) and the nucleus pulposus as a hard rubber tire (AF) and an inner tube (NP). Sometimes the tire splits and the inner tube pushes out. This occurrence is called a herniated disc (figure 2.5). The nerve fibers of the annulus fibrosa create a dull ache localized to the injured disc. A discogram, a procedure in which the disc is injected with liquid, uses the nerve fibers of the annulus fibrosa

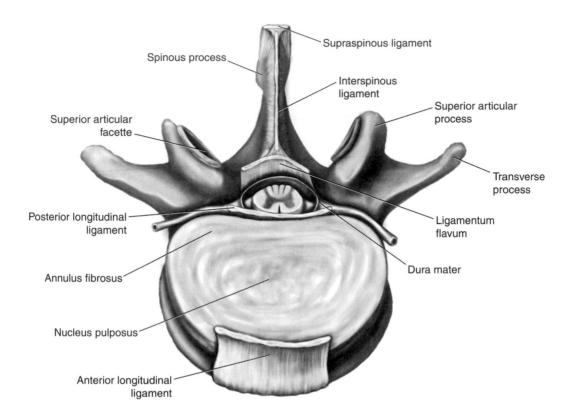

Figure 2.4 Vertebral disc.

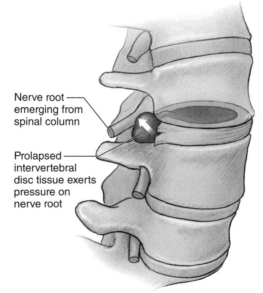

Figure 2.5 Herniated disc.

to indentify which disc is abnormal. If the injection of the liquid causes pain, that disc is abnormal. When the nucleus pulposus extrudes in a herniated disc, pressure can be put on the nerve root. This creates radicular pain, or radiculopathy (from *radice*, meaning "root," and *pathy*, meaning "suffering"). Therefore, radiculopathy means "suffering nerve root."

Myth

THE BULGING DISC REVEALED BY THE MRI MUST BE THE SOURCE OF MY PROBLEM

Technological advances have changed the way we live. Just as the cell phone made telegrams and phone booths obsolete, new technology has allowed some health care professionals to change the way in which they evaluate patients. These advances in technology have created a bit of a conundrum—helpful yet often confusing.

As technology has created better imaging tools, clinicians have become more dependent on using them to generate a primary diagnosis. Under increasing time constraints, physicians are doing more patient care in a smaller amount of time. An overreliance on imaging is the result. Dependence on these new technologies may lead us down the wrong path, confusing rather than clarifying a diagnosis.

A 1982 study reported that this new technology was not as effective as previously thought. Rather than enhancing the accuracy for specific diagnoses, it often did the opposite. The study revealed that patients over 50 years old without any complaints of pain were diagnosed with significant spinal disease 50 percent of the time because of MRIs. Some patients only 25 years old were diagnosed with significant spinal changes in 20 percent of the cases reviewed.

More recent studies also show the common nature of cervical and lumbar disc bulges across all segments of the population whether they are symptomatic or not. Disc bulges are a common finding, and imaging is only one part of the diagnostic process. If the imaging results do not support your history and physical exam, the chances of a correct diagnosis are poor.

LIGAMENT PAIN

The spine has several ligaments (figure 2.6). The anterior and posterior longitudinal ligaments are mainly for support. These ligaments are poorly innervated, which means that they give little pain but are anatomically important. When the disc space is normal size, these ligaments are stretched out. But as the disc dehydrates, which starts to occur after age 25, the disc begins to shrink, reducing the tautness of the ligaments and causing the ligaments to buckle, decreasing the size of the canal.

As we age, we lose height due to de-hydration of the nucleus pulposus and the collapse of a disc space. The buckling ligament goes into the central canal and can create narrowing, causing spinal stenosis (*stenosis* means "narrowing"; figure 2.7). In the neck, spinal stenosis puts pressure on the spinal cord and can result in paralysis or weakness from the neck down, a real medical emergency. If the narrowing occurs in the lumbosacral spine, you might lose strength in both legs.

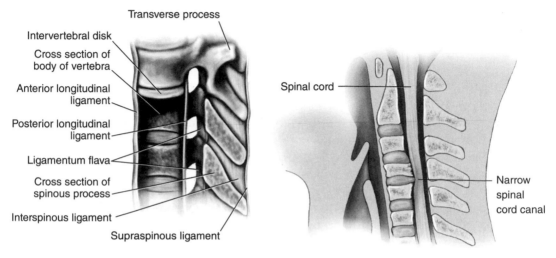

Figure 2.6   Ligaments of the spine.   **Figure 2.7**   Spinal stenosis.

SPINAL CORD INJURY

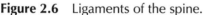

The spinal cord carries all the pain, motor, and coordination fibers of the body but does not have any pain receptors itself to speak of. What it does not say in pain, it says in actions and sensations. Sensation and strength, together with bowel and bladder function, are turned off or severely impaired. An injury at the cervical level results in quadriplegia, weakness or paralysis of all four extremities. Spinal cord impairment is a medical emergency.

Spinal cord impairment may occur slowly over months or years. At first, only segmental sensory loss or motor loss occurs. This means loss of sensation below the level of the injury. A patient once reported that when she took a shower she couldn't feel the water below her waist. Soon afterward both legs weakened and she lost control of her ability to urinate. Symptoms such as this constitute a medical emergency. If you experience any of these symptoms, immediately go to the emergency room.

BONE PAIN

The vertebral bone has an outer shell called the periosteum, which has many pain nerve fibers. The inner part, the cancellous, is a network of dense calcium bridges that reinforce the outer bone covering. Inside the cancellous is the nutrition network

> ## Osteoporosis and Osteopenia
>
> The word *osteo* means "bone." Osteopenia (*penia* means "too little") is a condition in which there is too little bone. Osteoporosis (*porosis* means "porous") is a condition in which the bone has holes. Most spine fractures result from accidents or osteoporosis, which weakens the bone and predisposes it to compression fractures. About 750,000 spine fractures occur each year, 80 percent in postmenopausal women, and 250,000 hip fractures occur each year as well.

that keeps the bone healthy. The inner cancellous has no nerves, so when injured it does not give the sensation of pain.

The quality of bone pain is severe, sharp, and localized over the injured bone. The onset of symptoms is usually sudden. The quantity is usually a 7 to 10 on a scale of 1 to 10. Lying down, bending, and twisting make the pain worse. Radiation is local and does not extend down the arm or leg unless the fracture compresses a nerve.

Bone pain is an acute, piercing pain localized to the area of the fracture; 60 percent of fractures occur to the thoracic 12 (T12) or L1 bones. Localization of pain often is over the spinous process, the steeple of the spine. Lying down makes pain worse, whereas sitting up makes it somewhat better. Bending, lifting, or twisting causes acute pain. Injury to the bone often is associated with secondary muscle spasm in the area. Bone pain is always a danger sign for possible severe spinal disease, such as severe osteoporosis or, rarely, a spinal tumor.

An immediate X-ray and medical evaluation is of utmost importance. Bone pain does not have sensory loss or motor loss or loss of bowel or bladder function, unless it causes narrowing and puts pressure on the spinal canal. In those with osteoporosis, fractures can occur without any acute trauma, such as a fall or an accident.

PSYCHOLOGICAL PAIN

Often the brain is not included as part of the anatomy of the spine, but it is a major contributor to all pain, especially chronic pain that lasts more than six weeks. Extensions from the brain, called axons, reach into the spine. All doctors know that without the brain, there is no pain. For that reason, doctors anesthetize people before any surgical procedure. Putting the brain to sleep puts pain to sleep. But the brain's appreciation of pain is great.

Any health care professional will tell you that the brain has volume control when it comes to pain. Having a dull ache and stiffness in your back from a joint is one thing, but if your brain interprets it as a malignant tumor that will soon paralyze you, that dull ache takes on a new severity including dread, anxiety, and even panic. Most doctors and nurses can attest to this based on their own experiences during training. The psyche works overtime.

Psychological Pain Test

1. Do you experience pain 24 hours a day, 7 days a week?
2. Does your pain awaken you most nights?
3. Is pain ruining your life?
4. Have you lost a significant amount of time from work?
5. Do you think that no one can help?
6. Do you believe that your family does not appreciate how much you hurt?
7. Have doctors suggested to you that your pain is imagined?

If you answered yes to four or more questions, you have chronic pain or depression. See a competent pain specialist.

The psyche often is controlled by neurotransmitters such as dopamine, serotonin, neuradenaline, glutamine, gabamine, cytokinins, and many others. Cytokinis are not kind; these hormones are extremely painful. Kinins, postaglandins, leukotrenes, and other factors such as substance P can stimulate pain receptors in the skin and elsewhere, markedly increasing pain. The immediate injury is like a bomb blast; the release of the kinins is the radiation or fire damage afterward. Pain control must take both into account, as well as the psychological component.

When we note that the pain is in the brain, this is not to say that it is imagined, faked, or made up. The brain, especially the brain stem and spinal cord pathways, can modulate the perception of pain. Remember, pain is a conscious perception. Someone who is comatose, despite severe injury, does not feel it. Someone who is unconscious feels no pain. Again, this is the reason that patients are put to sleep before surgery. People who have been hypnotized or who use acupuncture may perceive no pain despite being operated on because neurotransmitters and hormones have been activated and deactivated.

SLEEPLESSNESS AND PAIN PERCEPTION

Any person with pain will tell you that after a good night's sleep, pain is less, but after a bad night's sleep, pain is worse. Why?

Serotonin, a neurotransmitter, and other neurotransmitters block pain perception in the thalamus, the middle part of the brain, and ascending pathways in the spinal cord. Serotonin is not like morphine. Serotonin actually reduces the pain messages received by the conscious brain, just as the valves of a shower increase or decrease the flow of water. Morphine dulls consciousness, whereas serotonin increases consciousness and the feeling of well-being. Norepinephrine, another neurotransmitter, has also been shown to decrease pain perception.

Research shows that pain perception can be reduced or increased 10-fold depending in part on the increase or decrease in serotonin. Students who received ethylamine, which depletes serotonin, complained of severe pain from walking to class.

The effectiveness of a pharmacological agent depends on its actions on the body's complex system of neurotransmitters and hormones. Serotonin and noradrenaline either decrease or increase pain perception. They act like a thermostat, cooling or heating pain perception, turning it up or down.

At night especially, you want your pain turned down. Unfortunately, this is when pain is naturally turned up. Antidepressants and selective serotonin reuptake inhibitors (SSRIs) were initially designed to treat depression, but because of their effect on increasing serotonin and norepinephrine they were found to decrease pain perception and are now a first-line defense in the fight against chronic pain. The advantage of these drugs is that they don't cause dependency. (See chapter 10 for more on using medication to treat spinal pain.)

Sleeplessness is rampant in the United States. Often sleeplessness is self-induced, although many suffer from sleep disorders such as sleep apnea. Sleep apnea interferes with the stages of sleep that replenish the stores of serotonin, norepinephrine, and other neurotransmitters. Obstructive sleep apnea is a major cause of chronic pain and fibromyalgia. If you snore, feel tired or have headaches when you awaken in the morning, fall asleep easily during the day, have high blood pressure, or are overweight, check with your medical professional to discuss if you might have sleep apnea.

Proper sleep of seven to eight hours is essential for pain control and neurotransmitter levels. Those neurotransmitters determine pain threshold. We can tell whether a patient will overreact to a needle puncture just by holding her or his hand. If it is cold and sweaty, it means that the alarm neurotransmitter, adrenaline, is high, which increases pain awareness. Adrenaline, a fight or flight neurotransmitter, increases the perception of any stimulus. When adrenaline is high, the pain threshold is low.

Those who have slept well and have high serotonin levels can tolerate a lot of pain. In fact, the brain is not receiving the pain message because serotonin and other neurotransmitters are blocking it. People with chronic pain often sleep poorly and consequently have low levels of serotonin. A low level of serotonin is associated

---

Sleep Test

1. I fear night time because of my pain.
2. I snore.
3. I awaken more tired than when I went to bed.
4. I get less than six hours of sleep per night.
5. I often fall asleep watching television or after dinner.
6. I have a waist size of 35 inches (88.9 cm) for a woman or 40 inches (101.6 cm) for a man or larger.
7. I have gained 15 pounds or more since I hurt myself.

If you answered yes to two or more questions or answered yes to snoring, you are in urgent need of sleep evaluation for your pain.

with depression and low levels of adrenaline. This makes the pain threshold low and pain perception high. This condition is particularly true for those who have chronic pain that lasts six weeks or more.

The average person needs seven hours of sleep, not just seven hours in bed. Because pain is often worse at night, many pain sufferers begin to dread bedtime. This condition can be treated with cognitive therapy and a doctor who specializes in sleep disturbance.

Helping Yourself

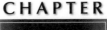

Using First Aid for Fast Relief

That moment before the pain starts can seem like an eternity. You know it's coming, from the moment you strike your finger with the hammer or stub your toe on the door, but it seems to take forever until you finally feel what you had expected. You might let out a yelp, say a choice word or two, or simply shake it off by wiggling your hand or foot. Gradually, the discomfort begins to disappear. No need to use ice, apply heat, tape it, soak it, or do anything really. It just gets better. Within two minutes you likely have forgotten the whole episode.

Why doesn't neck and lower back discomfort follow the same process? Why is discomfort in these areas often more difficult to resolve? Why does it linger? Why doesn't it just go away in the same short span as the pain fades from your smashed finger or stubbed toe?

If most back and neck issues were the result of a simple contusion, perhaps they too would resolve quickly and easily. But most spinal discomforts are not the result of an isolated bump or bruise. Rather, spinal pain more often arises from repeated wear and tear—long-term exposure to excessive stress and strain. When the discomfort is caused by a trauma such as a fall, sport, or an auto accident, multiple other factors influence the healing process. In these cases, we must consider the joints, muscles, discs, nerves, and ligaments as a whole, each having been stretched or compressed, twisted, or torn to varying degrees. This scenario is quite different from a simple bruise.

Because shaking it off is not feasible when dealing with neck or lower back pain, what can you do to ease the lingering and lasting discomfort that you feel? Read on to find out. This chapter is divided into two parts. First, we look at acute pain that follows a specific incident such as a fall, repetitive yard work, excessive overhead reaching, or a weekend of athletics. Second, we consider long-term discomfort that developed gradually and without apparent cause, has been present for some time, and is usually more annoying and frustrating than it is limiting.

Table 3.1 summarizes the self-care methods discussed in this chapter.

Table 3.1 Self-Care for Acute and Chronic Spinal and Neck Pain

	Acute pain	Chronic pain or stiffness
Cold application	Yes	Yes, for pain
Heat application	No	Yes, for stiffness
Activity	Avoid or minimize bed rest. Stay active within tolerance.	Modify activity to minimize aggravating factors. Assess body mechanics, workstation setup, and existing exercise program.
Cervical collar or lumbar corset	Use for short-term only for symptom relief. Avoid all day use.	Not recommended in most situations.
Medication	Over-the-counter anti-inflammatory drugs and pain reducers.	Based on your physician's recommendation. You must assess health risks with any long-term medication use.
Cervical pillow or lumbar roll	Useful.	Useful.
Exercise and conditioning	Not until you begin to feel improvement; then resume conservatively.	Recommended consistently for overall long-term health. Helps to minimize disuse atrophy and stimulates endorphins for long-term systemic pain relief.

SELF-TREATING ACUTE PAIN

Discomforts of this type generally limit movement and function. You may find it difficult to get out of bed, tie your shoes, brush your teeth, or sit to drive to work. You may not be able to easily stand and walk, lift your arm to get dressed, or turn your head to back out of the driveway.

When to Use Ice

Whenever you have pain or movement limitations, your immediate response should be to apply a cold pack. An acute injury always produces an associated inflammatory response. This inflammation leads to further pain, stiffness, and limited movement. Applying ice slows down local metabolism, thereby slowing the inflammatory reaction. By limiting the influx of cells known as leukocytes and slowing the release of inflammatory agents, you minimize the overall inflammatory process. The offending effects of the trauma can be reduced without the adverse effects of excessive swelling. In short, you'll heal faster and get back on your feet sooner.

For the first 72 hours following the injury, consistent application of a cold pack should be the intervention of choice. After that, continue using cold intermittently for as long as needed while the discomfort and mobility limitations persist. Initially, you'll want to keep icing to provide ongoing symptom relief and minimize the bleeding, swelling, and tissue trauma to the area around the injury. As you get better, you'll most likely begin to ice less, which is practical. Store bought reusable gel packs work well for the spine because they easily mold to the contours of the body.

⚠ Do not use a cold pack to treat spinal pain if you have an open or infected wound within the first 48 hours (this does not include a surgical incision that has been sutured closed, but rather an open cut or abrasion that has not yet begun to heal); skin hypersensitivity, which is rare for a spinal condition; or neurological conditions that compromise the vascular system or cause a loss of skin sensation.

Applying ice requires a balancing act of sorts. On the one hand, you want to ice long enough to cool the area and slow the inflammatory process. On the other hand, icing too long can create skin irritation. Most often, 15 to 20 minutes works best when using out-of-the-freezer reusable gel packs. The nice thing about gel packs is they warm slowly and eventually lose their cooling properties, limiting the possibility of skin irritation. Ice cubes tend to last a little longer and stay cold throughout the process, thereby requiring more attention to avoid skin problems. To minimize the likelihood of skin irritation, the best method is to place the cold or ice pack in a pillow case or over a piece of clothing (figure 3.1) rather than directly on your skin.

As a rule, you cannot apply a cold pack too many times in a day. If you're hurting and having difficulty moving, use a cold pack as often as you can, whether hourly or just once a day. You can apply the next cold pack as often as necessary as long as your skin has a chance to return to its normal color for at least 45 minutes before the start of the next 15- to 20-minute ice application.

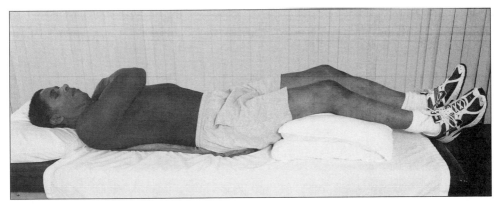

Figure 3.1   Applying a gel pack over clothing.

Why Not to Use Heat

Patients often ask about using heat or alternating between heat and cold. The recommended approach is to stick with cold for the duration of the acute period, about three weeks. Cold provides all the benefits that you're looking for in the initial healing stages of an injury—pain relief and reduced swelling. Combined, the result is improved mobility and function.

Myth

ALTERNATING HEAT WITH ICE IS HELPFUL FIRST AID

You just can't take it any longer. Seeking relief, do you choose an ice pack, a heat pack, or some combination? The basic rule is to use one or the other, depending on the situation. It is unnecessary and logistically cumbersome to alternate between them.

For example, if you have a recent injury with pain and presumed associated swelling, ice is the treatment of choice. Adding heat is counterproductive. If you have ongoing muscle stiffness or need help to loosen up before a tennis match, for example, heat is the treatment of choice. Ice is counterproductive. If persistent pain and end-of-the-day soreness is the issue, use ice. If you're stiff and need help working out the kinks, use heat.

Alternating back and forth is impractical. Both hot and cold packs tend to cool over time, so you'd have to have a second set ready for use after the first application. When you're trying to relax so that you can benefit from the heat or ice, the last thing you want to do is keep an eye on the timer to get up and switch the application after 10 minutes. By the time you get comfortable, it's time to change. This process is not practical when you're hurting.

Keeping it simple usually is the best medicine. In this case, base your choice on your situation and choose either heat or ice. It's not necessary to use both.

Alternating between heat and cold is a waste of time and effort. For acute injuries and pain, heat offers little value, and the task of alternating packs while keeping a fresh supply of both hot and cold is far too much work for someone trying to lie low and recuperate from an injury. This is not to say that a hot shower won't feel good. It most certainly could. But in terms of healing, stick with the cold or ice packs. You'll be glad that you did. We'll discuss the benefits of heat later in the chapter.

Get Up and Move

The second self-help remedy is to try to stay active. We now know that the recommendation to take two aspirin and stay in bed for a week is not the best advice. The medical literature is replete with information suggesting that long-term immobilization is counterproductive to healing. Most often, the quicker you resume or the longer you maintain your typical day-to-day activity, the faster you'll recover from whatever is ailing you. Consider, for example, the delivery person or the housewife. Neither may be able to lift and carry his or her usual amount for several days, but both can certainly stay involved with other tasks that prove useful and productive. When combined with the proper body mechanics that you'll learn in chapter 6, staying active minimizes muscle guarding, wards off muscle atrophy, and generally shortens your period of recuperation.

Certainly, wearing a neck brace, staying off your feet, or missing a day or two of work has merit at times. Giving an injured area a brief time to rest is advantageous. But make every attempt to continue your normal day-to-day activities as much as you can. You may have to give up sport practice, weekend tennis, lawn mowing, or recreational walks with the dog for a time, but keeping to as many of your usual activities as you can ensures that you're on the fast track to resuming all of them.

Study after study shows the advantages of staying active while recuperating from an injury or episode of pain. Many elements come into play during the recuperative period. Certainly, avoiding the bed rest trap is sound advice, but allowing yourself a short period of down time to get yourself together can be appropriate. A half day here or a missed day there when necessary is logical. Do not wait for the discomfort to abate completely before continuing with your life.

When to Use Devices and Accessories

Although cervical soft collars are sometimes useful, we avoid recommending them for all but specific conditions such as an acute fracture. A soft collar can provide a level of stability and comfort, especially after a trauma such as a motor vehicle accident or fall. Over time, however, they generally lead to poor cervical posture, promote weakness of the neck muscles, and limit mobility. If a soft collar gives you relief, by all means use one, but only for a short time. In the long term, avoid relying on them for comfort in place of therapy or some other health care intervention. As with any brace, soft collars do not replace the benefit of natural muscle support and therefore can be disadvantageous in the long run. We'll show you how to strengthen your muscles in chapter 4.

Similar in nature to cervical soft collars, lumbar corsets generally are recommended for short-term use when the injury first occurs or if existing discomfort flares up. Lumbar corsets are not intended as a long-term therapeutic option. The corset may make you feel better, which is beneficial in the short term, but no documented research shows that corsets themselves provide any functional external support or

---

The Case of Michelle

Michelle was a hard worker, but when she showed up at the doctor's office where she worked six hours early for her shift, the doctor knew that something was wrong. Michelle had injured her back at home when lifting one of her kids just two days before. She reported that she still could not move. It was painful to twist or bend to put on her shoes, and she could not easily get up from bed. Lifting her kids was out of the question. She was scheduled to work later that afternoon and wanted to know what to do. After a therapy session of back bends and ice, Michelle and the doctor agreed she would go to work and give it a try. She stayed busy doing what she could and reported steady progress by that evening. By the weekend, Michelle had resumed her usual activities both at home and at work.

prevent additional injury. Warehouse workers and delivery personnel often wear lumbar corsets, but their use in these situations poses some questions. True, a corset will help remind you of your spinal problem, perhaps encouraging better lifting technique and caution, but in real terms it will not make you any safer or stronger if you choose to wear one. If using one makes your back feel better in the short term, than use one. But do not rely on a corset to add any mechanical benefit after you are feeling better. That is a job for your trunk muscles. We'll describe what to do in chapter 4.

Recommending specific types of pillows or lumbar rolls is difficult. Many choices are available. Most work well for most people, and all of them work well for some people. Trying to identify who may benefit from one type or the other seems similar to offering an opinion on which shoe to buy; all may fit, but they will not all feel the same. Nevertheless, some general guidelines for choosing a neck pillow or lumbar roll may be helpful. Generally, spend less, not more. Because finding the right pillow or roll requires some trial and error, you may like a $20 roll as much as you do a $120 cushion. Also, think logically. If sleeping with your head flat on the bed aggravates your discomfort, then buying a pillow with a cutout in the middle for your head to rest in is probably not wise. If you routinely fall asleep while reading only to wake with neck pain, a tall, full, double thick pillow from a catalog is probably not for you. The same holds true for your back. Using a roll behind your back at work may be helpful, but chances are the chair you are sitting in can be adjusted to provide the same effect. And the $20 rolls work far better than the expensive cushions for travel, movies, and sporting events. Be conservative at first.

Pillows and cushions work because they promote a change in the resting position of the area where they are used. The change of position places whatever it is that is causing you discomfort in a different position—slackened, tensed, offset one way or another, and so on. In most cases, you can achieve a beneficial change of position using a less expensive item.

When to Use Medication

The third self-help intervention is over-the-counter medication. Acetaminophen, commonly packaged as Tylenol, is a fever reducer and pain reliever. It has no anti-inflammatory properties. Ibuprofen such as Motrin is an anti-inflammatory and offers symptom and fever relief as well. Naproxen, packaged as Aleve, also is an anti-inflammatory drug that offers pain and fever relief. Aspirin is an anti-inflammatory drug and pain reducer.

We recommend aspirin, ibuprofen, or naproxen in the doses prescribed on the label for immediate relief of pain and swelling associated with acute tissue trauma.

Muscle relaxers are another pharmaceutical option. Although not necessarily available as over-the-counter medication, muscle relaxers work to ease spasm and restore movement. They have no anti-inflammatory properties. Your doctor will advise you on the medications that he or she believes are best for you. For the best results, follow your doctor's advice because he or she is familiar with your medical history and the medications that you already use.

SELF-TREATING CHRONIC PAIN

Chronic discomforts of the spine or neck may be annoying and severely limiting. If you've had a recent flare-up of a long-term condition, please refer to the previous section on acute pain management. If you have chronic spinal pain that has not been aggravated recently, here are some basic self-intervention activities to help you feel better.

By definition, if your symptoms last longer than three months, you have chronic pain. Those with chronic discomfort have a unique set of dynamics to deal with. Many with chronic pain do not report abrupt activity limitations in the way that those with acute injuries or flare-ups do. Often chronic discomfort is described as a nagging stiffness, a deep aching, or an annoying and intensely frustrating feeling. It may be constant or intermittent, and it is usually not described as sharp, severe, or lancing.

Is It Pain or Stiffness?

If the complaint is pain, the recommendation will always be to use a cold pack. Often, however, chronic discomfort is accompanied by reports of stiffness and tightness that just won't go away. In these cases, heat may be appropriate. When muscle stiffness is the main complaint, a hot pack or heating pad likely will offer relief. Heat is the application of choice when stiffness and muscle soreness are the complaints.

Heat is advantageous because it comfortably promotes circulation to the area, thereby helping to flush the muscles of metabolic by-products that have built up over time from long-term muscle spasm. Reducing the chemical buildup in the muscle tissue can have a large effect on how you feel. True, a cold pack can accomplish this, too. But some people cannot fully relax onto a cold pack, thereby preventing the spasm from subsiding. In these cases heat is appropriate.

A typical time to stay on a heating pad or reusable hot pack is 20 minutes. You can use the heat as often as it is comfortable, so long as the skin has a chance to return to its normal color and temperature for at least 45 minutes before the next application. Obviously, the negative side effects are burns, some of which can be several layers deep if you're not careful. As a rule, avoid using the hot pad directly at bedtime and set a timer or alarm to alert you when 20 minutes has passed. Often the heat is soothing, and dozing off is not uncommon. Unfortunately, this is how burns occur.

Analyze Your Activities

For acute discomfort, maintain a level of activity that you can tolerate. For chronic discomfort, begin by analyzing your home and work environments to identify activities and positions that are aggravating. (See chapter 6 for body mechanics and chapter 7 for office workstation ergonomics.) Poor posture or movement habits may exacerbate the mechanism of your discomfort and keep the discomfort percolating. Immobilization over the long term is never the best answer. With chronic pain you will need to modify your activities and minimize those that exacerbate or increase the symptoms. We'll show you how in the chapters that follow.

Exercise and Conditioning

There is no magic pill, but properly prescribed and consistently done exercise comes close. Remember that not all exercises are right for every condition. A little common sense mixed with professional instruction can go a long way toward developing a program that is therapeutic rather than harmful. We'll discuss stretches and exercises in the next chapter. For now, suffice it to say in most chronic pain cases, performing a stretch and exercise regimen can at least ease discomfort. A regular program can go a long way toward helping you feel better and tolerate more during the week. Perhaps the best way to begin is by choosing activities that address your overall level of fitness. Walking, swimming, and using a stationary bike are three simple activities that begin the process of improving your fitness level and easing discomfort.

Sleep Well

Later in chapter 5 we'll discuss the effects of sleep on the body's healing and restorative process. Most chronic pain patients have some form of sleep loss which results in an escalation of their pain perception. The chemical serotonin acts as a pain dampener and is secreted in the deeper stages of sleep. Cortisol is serotonin's opposite, working to ramp up the perception of discomfort. Cortisol is secreted when you are anxious, tired, or angry, three common traits that chronic pain patients express. Coincidental? Not likely.

One way to promote a restful night's sleep is to avoid stimulants such as caffeine and chocolate late in the day. Turkey and dairy products such as milk and cheese tend to be useful late night snacks for promoting a good night's sleep.

Stretching is another way to help calm the body into a restful mode. As we'll discuss in chapter 4, long and soft stretches tend to be quieting to the nervous system, ramping down neurological input to help ease spasm and restrictive muscle pain. Stretches should be held for 60 seconds or longer and done two or three times each. The pull should be steady but conservative, well below symptom threshold. In most cases, stretching is the self-intervention that provides the most benefit for chronic pain sufferers. You can do all the stretches in designated sessions over the course of the day, or you can focus on the one or two that provide specific relief to your back or neck as often as necessary. In either case, you'll be surprised at how much relief some simple stretching can provide.

Whether you take over-the-counter medication, change your body mechanics, modify your activity, use a lumbar belt or cervical soft collar for a brief period, begin some stretching activities, or use a hefty dose of ice for a time, you can get some immediate symptom relief through your own actions.

The point of this chapter is not to imply that eliminating your discomfort is simple. Obviously, that is not the case. Use this information to begin the healing process and start moving toward restoring your body's ability to carry on without limitation.

CHAPTER

4

Stretching and Exercising

Stretches and exercises are two of the best ways to relieve and prevent spinal pain. No one program will fit everyone's needs, but the recommendations in this chapter offer you an excellent opportunity to make progress in reducing your discomfort. You can do these exercises and stretches at home without any elaborate or expensive equipment. Because they are slow, low-resistance exercises, they minimize the likelihood of injury. These exercises and stretches are time and patient tested, producing successful results for patients of all ages and physical ability.

We rely on two specific types of exercise programs and a variety of stretches. The primary exercise program is a trunk stabilization and chest-out posturing regimen. The second program is an isometric routine. You will find additional suggestions and caveats for gym-based programs toward the end of the chapter.

TRUNK STABILIZATION

The technique for all stabilization exercises is generally the same. The trunk stabilization program focuses on exercises performed in a variety of positions and different intensity levels to accommodate individual skill. The addition of arm movement, leg movement, or both adds difficulty to the exercise, but the basic trunk muscle contraction remains the same. The level of difficulty is always presented from easy to more difficult.

In all cases, the goal is to find the spinal position of maximum comfort or least discomfort in which the spine is neither fully flexed nor fully extended, a position referred to as the neutral position. By exercising in the neutral position, you train the muscles to support your spine and maintain the position most conducive to feeling better.

Stabilization training produces a coordination of trunk muscle function. Coordinated strength is more effective than uncoordinated strength because training teaches each of the trunk muscles to fire in a precise sequence for a particular activity. This coordinated strength protects the spine from injury and improves your ability to complete day-to-day, recreational, and athletic activities without discomfort.

The key is to learn the proper technique. Unlike strength training at a gym, stabilization training does not require brute force. Initially, these are finesse exercises, requiring you learn the technique properly and progress through increasing levels of difficulty. By the time you reach the upper level, your muscles will be well conditioned to tolerate the activities that you need or would like to do.

Trunk stabilization requires a cocontraction of the torso muscles. This action requires the abdominals and paraspinous muscles (semispinalis, iliocostalis, multifidus—the neck and back extensors) to hold your spine in the position of relative comfort that you choose. To find the position of comfort, arch and flatten your lower back until you find the spot that gives the most comfort or the least discomfort. The concept is the same for lower back, midback, or neck discomfort, making a stabilization program appropriate for spinal discomfort regardless of location.

To achieve the proper contraction, think of the feeling that you get when your abdominal muscles tighten just as you begin to sneeze. Mothers may be able to relate to the feeling of pushing during labor. Men may have better luck imagining tightening their abdomen as if to absorb a pending blow. Picture your rib cage moving down toward your feet. Don't suck in and don't push your abdomen out. Rather, bear down as if to show off your six-pack. They're in there. Sometimes they just need a little coaxing to come out.

Whether you are lying on your back, lying on your belly, kneeling on your hands and knees, or standing, your spine should remain in the position of greatest comfort for the full duration of the exercise. During the exercise, your spine should neither arch nor sag when you contract the trunk muscles. After you've found the spot of relative comfort, tighten those muscles by moving the ribs toward the feet and hold. A good cue is to simulate a good hearty sneeze.

To help you feel the contraction, place the tips of your fingers on the lower abdomen, just above the belt line about halfway from the navel to your sides (figure 4.1). You should feel the muscles harden beneath the tips of your fingers if you're doing it right.

After the muscles have been activated, keep them on throughout the exercise. The goal is to maintain the basic trunk cocontraction throughout the exercise, especially when adding difficulty by moving your arms and legs. Attempt to maintain the contraction for two consecutive minutes at a time. After this is easy, increase the difficulty by adding time or by progressing to the next stabilization exercise. The ability to complete the exercise without arching or flattening your back for two minutes is the sign that you are ready to move to the next level.

The simple and straightforward exercises in this section cover a lot of therapeutic ground, providing relief for most patients. Even so, we provide only the first level or two for many exercises. As exercises become more complicated, the chance for error increases, which can potentially undo the benefits. Often maintaining a simple program that is working is more advantageous than progressing to harder activities. This routine has enough room to add difficulty without compromising safety.

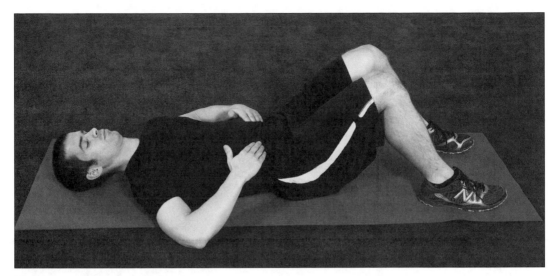

Figure 4.1   Feel the trunk contract.

! The activities in this chapter are presented as guidelines for self-help. In general, these exercises are safe for a variety of conditions of various severities and are not likely to cause additional harm. If an exercise hurts, that is, if it causes an increase in discomfort that does not quickly subside after you've stopped the activity, you may not be doing the activity correctly or it may not be the right exercise for you. Try again over the next two or three days to work on your technique, but if the discomfort still increases then stop. Be sure to differentiate your pain from the soreness that comes with doing new activities.

SELF-CARE ACTIVITIES FOR POSTURAL SYNDROME

This section covers activities specific to the postural syndrome. In these situations, discomfort is always local to the structure causing the symptoms and is intermittent in nature. It is seldom severe or debilitating. Common descriptive terms are annoying, nagging, and gnawing, but not intense or urgent. If your symptoms are postural related, exercise is the primary intervention. By definition, flexibility is not limited.

Postural syndrome diagnoses include headaches, neck pain, cervical strain, midscapular pain, thoracic strain, low back pain, and lumbar strain. Generally, these diagnoses are vague because there often is little clinical finding of a medical or pathological nature.

Postural Exercises

Choose one activity within each group or choose five or six exercises to perform. Each activity should be performed for two consecutive minutes at a time. Although a daily dosage might be best, reality dictates the likelihood of performing the exercises three or four times a week. More would be fine, especially if they help you feel better. To get off to a good start, commit to three or four times a week. More advanced exercises are indicated by an asterisk.

Supine

Bracing With Arm Flexion

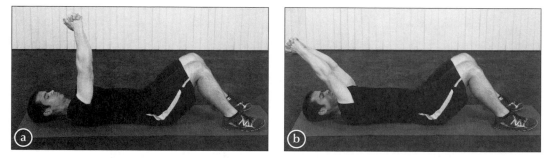

Lie on your back. Contract your trunk muscles using the technique described on page 46. After you've found the position of maximum comfort, clasp your hands together (a) and move your arms back and forth at a comfortable pace (b). Avoid arching your back. Maintain the contraction for two consecutive minutes. To make the exercise more difficult, hold a 5- to 10-pound (2.3 to 4.5 kg) weight.

Bracing With Leg Extension

Lie on your back. As in bracing with arm flexion, contract your trunk muscles using the technique described on page 46 to find the position of maximum comfort (a). Kick one leg out (b) and return it to the starting position before kicking the other leg out. Slowly and softly set your foot on the floor after the kick and before you switch to the other leg. Avoid arching your back. Maintain the contraction for two consecutive minutes.

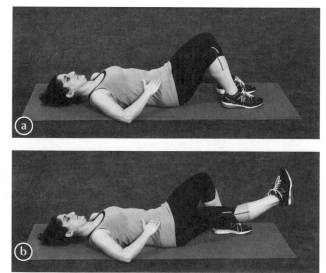

Unsupported Bracing*

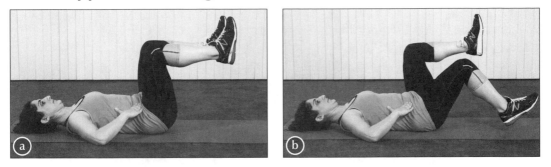

Lie on your back. As in bracing with arm flexion, contract your trunk muscles using the technique described on page 46. Move your legs to the starting position as shown in *a*. Slowly lower one foot, softly tapping the heel on the ground (*b*), and then return to the starting position. Lower the other foot the same way. Avoid arching your back. Maintain the contraction for two consecutive minutes.

Partial Curl-Up

Lie on your back with your legs straight and your arms pointing toward the ceiling (*a*). Contract your trunk muscles until in the position of maximum comfort using the technique described on page 46. Tuck your chin as you reach up, moving your forehead, chest, and hands toward the ceiling (*b*). Maintain the contraction even as you lower back to the starting position. The trunk muscles contract the entire time. Avoid letting them relax. Repeat, reaching up again. Do as many as you can while keeping your chin tucked and abdominal muscles activated. When you cannot complete the motion with proper technique, stop and rest. A typical set is 5 to 15 repetitions.

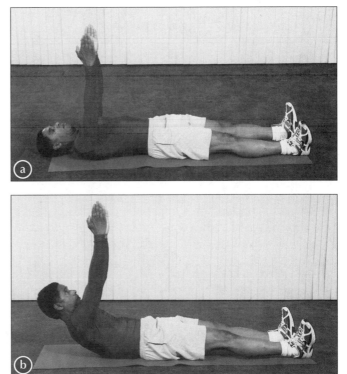

*Advanced exercise.

Partial Curl-Up With Twist*

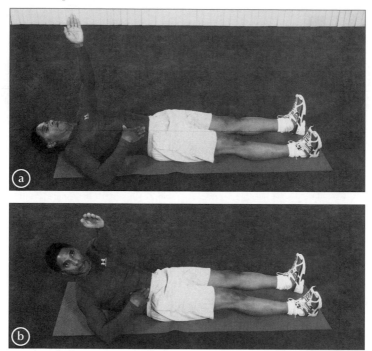

Lie on your back with your legs straight. Lift your left arm, pointing the hand toward the ceiling, and rest your right hand on your torso (a). Contract your trunk muscles once in the position of maximum comfort using the technique described on page 46. Tuck your chin as you reach up and then twist slightly to the right (b). Return to the starting position and repeat 5 to 10 times. Switch arms, pointing your right hand toward the ceiling and placing your left hand on your torso, and repeat to the left. Keep your abdominal muscles activated throughout the entire exercise set.

Bridging

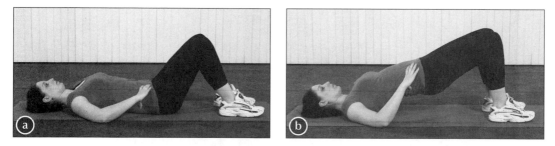

Lie on your back with your knees bent, feet flat on the floor and close to your buttocks, and arms by your sides, hands on your hips (a). Find your position of maximal comfort. Press your heels into the floor and lift your hips toward the ceiling (b). Be sure to move your ribs and hips at the same time in one block. Avoid tucking your hips under or arching your back. Lift as high as you can without arching your back. Lower to the floor and repeat. Focus on contracting your buttock muscles and moving the ribs and hips as one block. The goal is to continue the exercise for two consecutive minutes.

Bridging With Leg Extension*

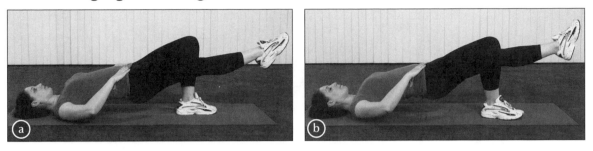

Lie on your back with your knees bent and your feet flat on the floor close to your buttocks as in the bridging exercise. Place your hands on your hips. After lifting your hips and ribs in one block, kick one leg out (a), return it to the ground, and then kick the other leg out (b). Resist dropping or swaying your hips when you balance on just one leg. Firmly press down with the heel into the floor when you begin to pick the opposite foot off the ground and slowly and softly place the foot back on the ground. The goal is to continue the exercise for two consecutive minutes.

> ⚠ If you think that an exercise may not be quite right for you, likely it is the bridge exercise. Withhold the bridge and analyze how you feel. Periodically try to resume the exercise as your symptoms allow.

*Advanced exercise.

Hands and Knees

Quadruped Transverse Abdominals

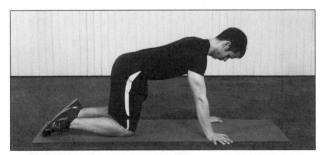

Get on your hands and knees. Find your position of maximum comfort. Without moving, lift your lower abdomen, the area below your navel, toward your spine. Do not arch your upper back. You should feel the lowest part of your abdomen working. Do not suck in. Concentrate on lifting the area below your navel toward the spine. To help you find the right contraction, tighten the pelvic floor muscles at the same time. No observable motion should occur. Hold the contraction for 10 to 20 seconds, relax, and repeat. The goal is to accumulate two minutes of contraction time, so do 12 reps if you hold each contraction for 10 seconds or 6 reps if you hold each contraction for 20 seconds.

Modified Plank

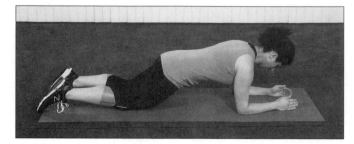

Get on your forearms and knees and have your feet on the ground. Without moving, lift your lower abdomen, the area below your navel, toward your spine. Do not arch your upper back. You should feel the lowest part of your abdomen working. Do not suck in. Concentrate on lifting the area below your navel toward the spine. To help you find the right contraction, tighten the pelvic floor muscles as if trying to stop urinating. No observable motion should occur. Hold the contraction for 10 to 20 seconds, relax, and repeat. The goal is to achieve two minutes of contraction time, so do 12 reps if you hold each contraction for 10 seconds or 6 reps if you hold each contraction for 20 seconds.

Plank*

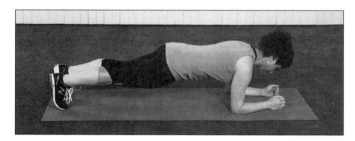

Get on your forearms and tip toes. Without moving, lift your lower abdomen, the area below your navel, toward your spine. Do not arch your upper back. You should feel the lowest part of your abdomen working. Do not suck in. Concentrate on lifting the area below your navel toward the spine. To help you find the right contraction, tighten the pelvic floor muscles as if trying to stop urinating. No observable motion should occur. This difficult exercise places a lot of strain on the spine. Start with just a few repetitions and assess how you feel.

*Advanced exercise.

Prone

Prone Transverse Abdominals

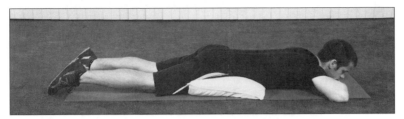

Lie on your belly. Place a pillow under your hips if it feels better. Find the position of maximum comfort as you lift your lower abdominals, the area below your navel, toward your spine. Your hips and midback should not move at all. To help you find the right contraction, tighten the pelvic floor muscles as if you are trying to stop urinating. No observable motion should occur. Hold the contraction for 10 to 20 seconds, relax, and repeat. The goal is to achieve two minutes of contraction time, so do 12 reps if you hold each contraction for 10 seconds or 6 reps if you hold each contraction for 20 seconds.

Prone Transverse Abdominals With Leg Lift

Lie on your belly. Place a pillow under your hips if it feels better. Find the position of maximum comfort as you lift your lower abdominals, the area below your navel, toward your spine. Your hips and midback should not move at all. To help you find the right contraction, tighten the pelvic floor muscles as if you are trying to stop urinating. Without arching your back, slowly lift one leg off the floor, keeping the knee straight (a). Lift from the hip, using your buttock muscle. Your knee should not bend, and your back should not arch. Lift only a small distance. Slowly lower and repeat with the other leg (b). The goal is to continue the exercise for two consecutive minutes.

Prone Transverse Abdominals With Arm Lift*

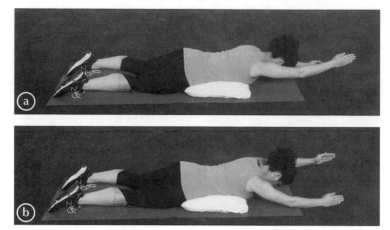

Lie on your belly. Place a pillow under your hips if it feels better. Find the position of maximum comfort as you lift your lower abdominals, the area below your navel, toward your spine. Your hips and midback should not move at all. To help you find the right contraction, tighten the pelvic floor muscles as if you are trying to stop urinating. Without arching your back, slowly lift one arm off the floor (a). Keep your head in the starting position; avoid looking up. Lift only a small distance. Slowly lower your arm and repeat with the other arm (b). Feel your abdominals and midback muscles working. The goal is to continue for two consecutive minutes.

Seated

Seated Arm Lift

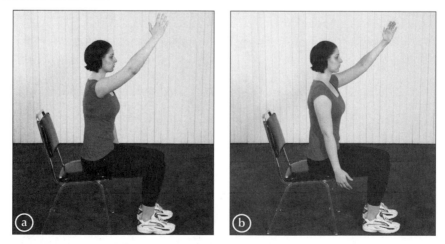

Sit on a sturdy chair with your arms at your sides. Find the position of maximum comfort and contract your trunk muscles as described on page 46. Slowly lift one arm toward the ceiling (a), return it to the starting position, and then lift the other arm (b). Avoid arching your back or leaning back. Stretch and elongate, reaching up toward the ceiling, trying to make yourself tall. The goal is to continue the exercise for two consecutive minutes.

Seated Arm and Leg Lift*

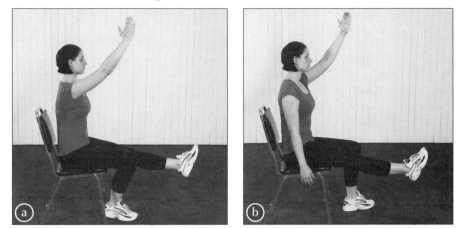

Sit on a sturdy chair with your arms at your sides. Find the position of maximum comfort and contract your trunk muscles as described on page 46. Slowly lift one arm toward the ceiling. As you stretch the arm toward the ceiling, kick the opposite leg out in front of you (a). Slowly return the arm and leg to the starting position and repeat with the other arm and leg (b). Move slowly and avoid leaning, slumping, or arching the trunk. Remember to make yourself tall. The torso moves minimally or not at all as you slowly alternate moving the arms and legs. The goal is to continue the exercise for two consecutive minutes.

Standing

Sumo Position Arm Lift

Stand with your feet wider than hip-width apart and your toes pointing straight ahead. Be careful to keep the weight on your heels and your head looking forward, not down. The knees should be slightly bent. Hold this position as you slowly lift one arm forward, thumb up (a), and return it to the starting position. Then lift the other arm (b). The arms should be the only part moving. Continue the exercise for two minutes. You may add weights as tolerated.

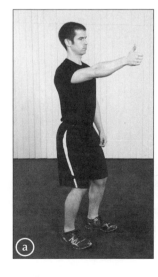

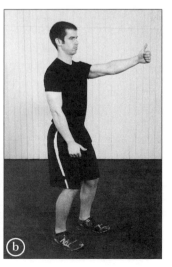

*Advanced exercise.

Sumo Position Lateral Raise

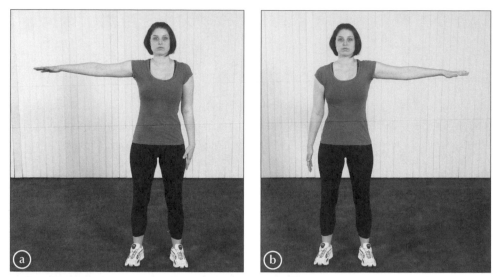

Stand with your feet wider than hip-width apart and your toes pointing straight ahead. Keep the weight on your heels and look forward, not down. The knees should be slightly bent. Hold this position as you slowly lift one arm out to the side (a), return it to the starting position, and then lift the other arm (b). Alternate sides, continuing the exercise for two minutes. You may add weights as tolerated.

Ball Exercises

Supine Bridge to Partial Curl*

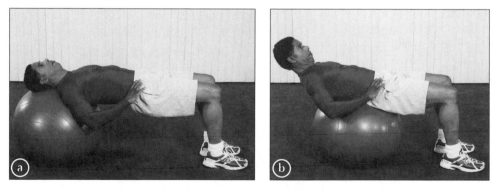

Lie face up on the exercise ball. Maintain this position as you move on the ball from the bridge (a) to the partial curl (b). Place your hands at your hips for the bridge. Try to hold each position for 15 to 20 seconds and perform each exercise for two minutes.

Prone Leg Extension to Plank*

Lie face down on the exercise ball. Maintain this position, moving on the ball from the leg extension (a) to the plank (b). Keep the upper legs together for both exercises. Do not allow the legs to drop during the leg extension and keep your back from sagging toward the floor during the plank. Try to hold each position for 15 to 20 seconds and perform each exercise for two minutes.

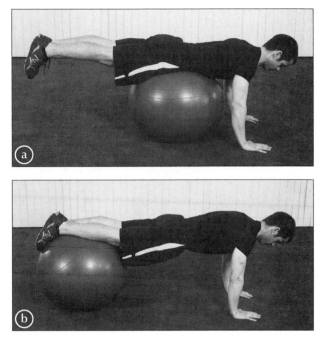

Chest-Out Exercises for Midscapular and Cervical Pain

An effective exercise program for self-treating common neck and upper thoracic pain should include the postural exercises covered in the previous section as well as selected exercises from this section. A well-rounded program for the trunk will include one exercise from each of the position categories.

It is easy to understand why chest-out posturing affects your neck. Look in a mirror. Intentionally slouch, allowing your upper back to hunch forward and your shoulders to round to the front. Your head will follow in a predictable pattern, eyes gazing forward while the neck compresses in the back. Now stand upright, chest up and out, shoulder blades slightly back. What happens to the position of your neck? Does it feel less compressed, less compacted? It should. A chest-out posture puts the head in proper alignment on the neck. As you slouch, your neck compresses posteriorly, setting you up for a variety of symptoms.

*Advanced exercise.

Standing

Rowing

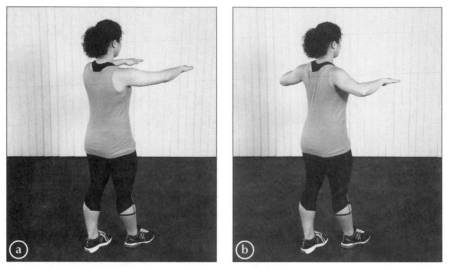

Stand with your feet slightly staggered, knees slightly bent, and torso upright as if you were balancing a book on your head (*a*). Pull your elbows back, pinching the shoulder blades as if rowing a boat (*b*). Palms stay turned down to the floor. Hold for five counts, return to the starting position, and repeat. The goal is two minutes of exercise time.

External Rotation

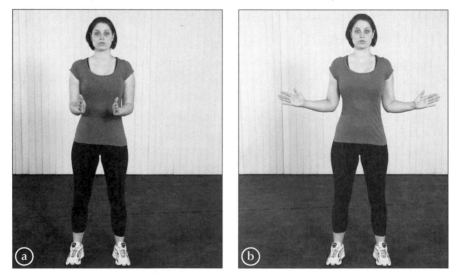

Stand with your feet shoulder-width apart, knees slightly bent, and torso upright as if you were balancing a book on your head (*a*). Rotate your forearms out, keeping the elbows firmly against your sides and the thumbs up (*b*). Pinch the shoulder blades and move your chest forward as the arms move out. Hold for five counts, return to the starting position, and repeat. The goal is two minutes of exercise time.

Prone

Neck Retraction*

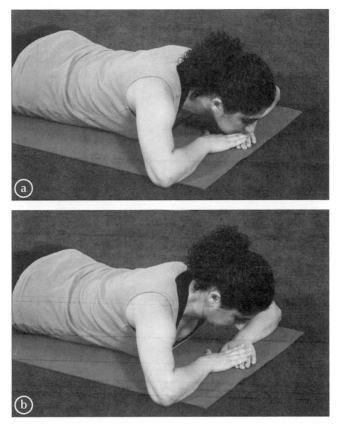

Lie on your abdomen (a). You may lie with your head hanging over the edge of a bed or your chest resting on a pillow. Move your chin up and away from the floor (b). You should not look up. Instead, emphasize moving the back of your head straight up, moving the chin away from the floor. Your upper back may come off the floor a little. Hold for five counts, return to the starting position, and repeat. The goal is two minutes of exercise time.

CARDIOVASCULAR CONDITIONING

Cardiovascular conditioning is a key component to any overall fitness program. This topic will be covered more fully in chapter 5. The goal is to perform at least 20 minutes of consecutive cardiovascular activity while keeping your heart rate in your training zone. Varying the training activity is important to minimize overuse injury and work different parts of the body. Common cardiovascular exercises are walking, biking, light jogging or running, swimming, using a stationary arm bike, or training on an elliptical machine. Calculate your target heart rate (see page 83) and determine your cardiovascular training zone before you start.

*Advanced exercise.

SELF-CARE ACTIVITIES FOR ADAPTIVE SHORTENING SYNDROME

The primary component of adaptive shortening syndrome, also called dysfunction syndrome, is a loss of motion. Self-help for this condition begins with flexibility and then strengthening. The key is to ease compression by elongating shortened muscles and connective tissues with gentle but consistent stretching. All stretches should be held for at least 30 seconds, preferably for 60 seconds or more. Perform each stretch several times a day. The quality of stretching depends on how often you do it and how long you hold it, not how hard you stretch. A stretch with a long, soft hold is more beneficial than a brief, hard stretch. Although initially stretching is key, strengthening is also important. When choosing a mix of activities, rely first on several stretches and one or two exercises. Gradually add to your program until you have about equal time for each. As you improve, adjust the routine to a combination of activities that you like and find useful.

Adaptive shortening syndrome diagnoses may include headaches; neck, mid-thoracic, or low back pain; cervical, thoracic, or lumbar strain; cervical or lumbar stenosis; radiculopathy; sciatica; degenerative joint disease; facet arthropathy; thoracic outlet syndrome; or myofascial pain syndrome.

Remember to start with stretches. As you feel better, add more exercises to your program. By definition, adaptive shortening symptoms reflect a shortening of muscles and connective tissue. Therefore, stretching is the initial line of defense in a self-help program and should make up at least 75 percent of your self-help effort the first few weeks. As you begin to feel better add exercises for a 50–50 mix.

Neck and Upper Back Stretches

Neck patients often benefit from exercises that stretch the front of the chest and the chest-out posturing exercises covered on page 57. Often neck retraction is useful. Retraction involves gliding the head straight back, keeping your eyes focused on the same spot, and not moving the chin up or down.

Seated or Standing

Neck Muscles: Trapezius

Either sit in a chair or stand. Place one arm behind your back, allowing it to rest gently behind you. Avoid holding the arm up. Instead, let it rest freely and hang to pull the shoulder blade down. Move your head to the side, using the other arm to apply a small amount of pressure. Do not rotate your head. Keep your nose pointing straight forward. Hold the head to the side for one minute. Repeat two times on both sides before moving to the next stretch. The goal is two minutes of stretch time for each side.

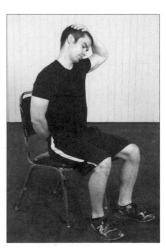

Neck Muscles: Levator

Either sit in a chair or stand. Place one arm behind your back, allowing it to rest gently behind you. Avoid holding the arm up. Instead, let it rest freely and hang to pull down the shoulder blade. Move your head toward the opposite hip, using the other arm to apply a gentle amount of pressure. Move the chin and nose toward the hip. To stretch the right side, move the nose toward the left hip; to stretch the left side, move the nose toward the right hip. Hold the head in the stretch position for one minute. Repeat two times on both sides and then move to the next stretch. The goal is two minutes of stretch time for each side.

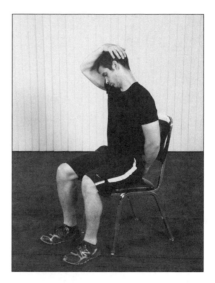

Neck Muscles: Scalene

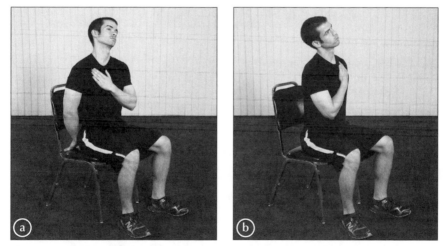

Sit in a chair or stand. Place your right arm behind your back, allowing it to rest gently behind you. Avoid holding the arm up. Instead, let it rest freely and hang to pull down the shoulder blade. Move your head to the left and slightly back, as if looking up and slightly off center. Place the left hand on the front of your chest and apply a slight downward pressure (a). This will help stretch the front of your neck on the opposite side as the hand that is pressing down on your chest. You should feel a pull along the front side of your neck. Switch sides (b). Note that the hand placements have changed from the first two stretches. The goal is two minutes of stretch time for each side.

Standing

Sun Salutation

Sit or stand in a fully upright position. Reach overhead as high as you can (a). Turn your palms forward and move your elbows firmly down toward your back pockets (b). Pinch your shoulder blades together. Hold for five counts and repeat from the starting position. The goal is two minutes of exercise time.

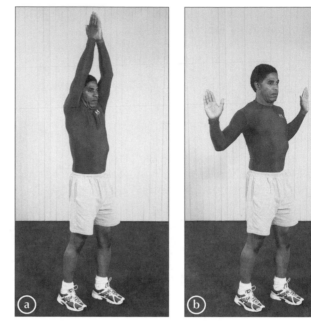

Front of Chest Stretch

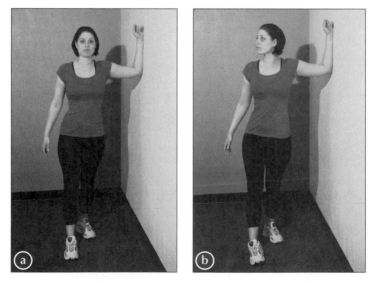

Stand with your feet staggered and your forearm against a wall or door frame (a). Position yourself so that a slight twist away from the side that you are stretching (b) produces a pull along the front of your chest. Hold for up to 60 counts. Switch sides and stretch the other side. The goal is two minutes of stretch time on each side.

Upper Back Mobility

Stand facing a wall with your feet staggered (a). Slide your hands up the wall, allowing your upper back to sag as you move closer to the wall (b). Your head should follow your hands so that you are looking up as you near the end of the movement. Hold for 10 to 20 counts per repetition. The goal is two minutes of stretch time.

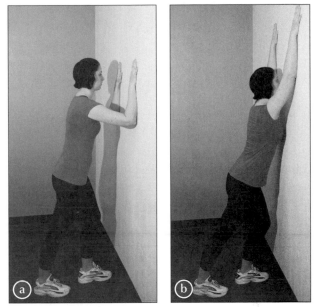

Supine

Elongate

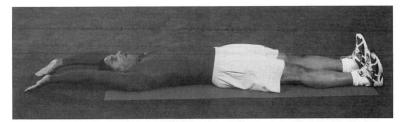

Lie on your back with your arms stretched over your head and your legs straight. Stretch your torso by moving your heels in one direction while reaching the hands in the other direction. Try to get long, elongating your trunk as best you can. The goal is to stretch yourself as your arms and legs move in opposite directions away from the middle. Hold for 30 counts per repetition. The goal is two minutes of stretch time.

Lower Back and Hip Stretches

When combined with stabilization exercises, activities that stretch the lower back and the front of the hip will help ease low back discomfort. If you have lower back issues, you may have heard that your problem is tight hamstrings. It used to be that everyone with a lower back problem was thought to have tight hamstrings in need of stretching. We understand now that this is not the case. Many years ago, Donna came to physical therapy with a deep ache in her leg. The diagnosis was sciatica.

Her newly trained therapist gave her a hamstring stretch to address the tightness uncovered during the evaluation. We've come to understand that Donna's tightness was not in the muscle but rather was a symptom of an irritated nerve root. Stretching was not the right treatment for Donna, and she did not come back because the stretching significantly irritated the already inflamed nerve root.

In a similar way, arm pain was often said to be caused by tight neck muscles, and neck stretches were thought to help. This is true sometimes, but not always. If you have deep bandlike arm or leg pain, often described as a pulling or tightness, be sure to keep your knee slightly bent or your arm on your lap when you begin any hamstring or neck stretch. Evaluate the stretch for usefulness. Proceed conservatively, keeping the knee bent if you have leg symptoms or the hand on your lap if you have arm symptoms. This will keep the nerve root slack to soften the nerve root tension. Shorten the hold to 20 seconds and apply a gentle, conservative stretch until you're confident that the stretching feels good. A well-trained therapist can show you the best positions for you.

Supine

Lower Trunk Rotation

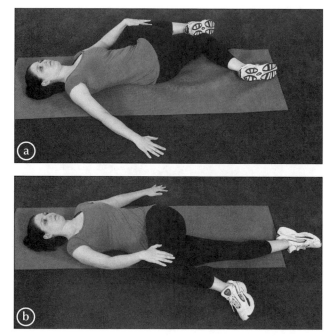

Lie on your back. Roll both knees to one side. Use the arm to pull the top knee across until you feel a stretch across your lower back (a). You may have to adjust the bottom leg, usually back, to find a stretch that feels good across your lower back. Hold for up to 30 counts then switch sides (b). The goal is two minutes of stretch time in each direction.

! If you have a total hip replacement, avoid pulling the leg with the replacement across your body. In this case, focus on twisting your lower back and minimize pulling the leg across.

Outer Hip Stretch

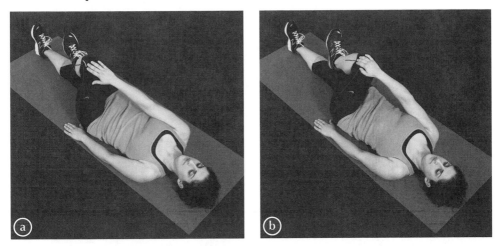

Lie on your back. Place the heel of one foot just above the knee of the opposite leg (*a*). Use your hand to pull the knee softly across (*b*), being careful not to let your back move off the floor. Only the knee should be pulled across. After your back starts to roll as well, stop and hold the stretch for up to 30 counts. The goal is two minutes of stretch time on each side.

> **!** If you have a total hip replacement, avoid pulling the leg with the replacement across your body. In this case, do not perform this stretch on the side of the hip replacement. Performing this stretch on the other side is fine.

Seated

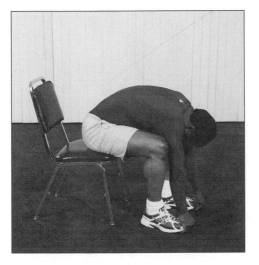

Lower Back Flexion Stretch

Sit at the edge of a chair. Move your trunk forward and reach down to your feet. You may move either over your knees as shown or between your knees. If you have a hip replacement, move between your knees. Hold for 30 counts. The goal is two minutes of stretch time.

Kneeling

Hip Flexor Stretch

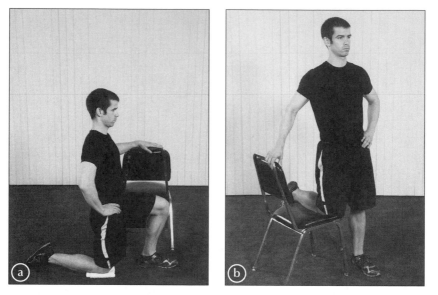

Assume a half-kneeling position (a). If kneeling is a problem, stand as shown in b. In either case, have an object nearby to hold onto to help with balance. Tuck your hips under and shift your weight forward slightly until you feel a pull across the front of your thigh. Hold for 30 to 60 counts and then switch sides. Repeat to reach the goal of two minutes of stretch time on each side.

Standing

Heel Cord Stretch

Stand and place one foot on a small platform (towel roll, tree root, rock, two by four, block, small ball). Stretch the calf of your back leg by slightly shifting your weight forward onto the front foot. Hold for 30 to 60 counts and then switch legs. The goal is two minutes of stretch time on each side.

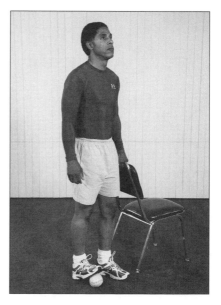

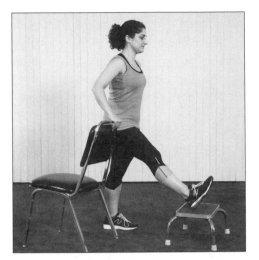

Hamstring Stretch

Stand and place one foot on a sturdy object of a manageable height, such as a chair, park bench, or bleacher step. While holding onto a nearby object for balance, rotate your hips back so that you feel a stretch along the back of your elevated leg. You can keep your knee straight or bend it slightly, whichever feels best. Hold for 30 to 60 counts and then switch legs. The goal is two minutes of stretch time on each side.

SELF-CARE ACTIVITIES FOR DERANGEMENT SYNDROME

Derangement syndrome conditions most often affect people in the 25- to 50-year-old age group. Often they are the result of a flexion-biased lifestyle. These conditions elicit pain across the neck or back, into one shoulder blade or buttock, into one arm or leg, or all the way to the hand or foot. Bending and sitting often worsen the pain, while standing and walking often make it feel better. Getting up from a chair, bending to brush your teeth, putting on your shoes, lifting your arms above your head, or carrying things may be difficult. People often feel stiff in the morning. Symptoms typically ease by midday only to increase again by evening. Coughing, sneezing, reading, and computer work may increase discomfort and cause difficulty in turning the head, looking up, or bending forward.

Derangement syndrome diagnoses imply disc issues such as spondylosis, bulge, or herniation. Although not of the true McKenzie classification system, in this category we are also going to include those conditions with a disruption of normal tissue, such as a fracture. Therefore, we include diagnoses of spondylolisthesis and compression fractures along with disc bulges and herniations.

> ⚠️ Spondylolisthesis conditions require forward-bending stretches. Disc bulges and compression fractures benefit from back-bending activities. Do not mix the two. Repeated forward bending is counterproductive to discogenic issues and compression fractures, and repeated back bending is not appropriate for those with a diagnosis of spondylolisthesis or severe facette arthropathy. If repeated back bends or extension activities such as lying on your belly continually aggravate your symptoms, facette injections may provide great relief. (See chapter 11.)

Repeated Movement Activities

Disc bulges often respond favorably to repeated back bend and neck retraction exercises. The concept is to milk or maneuver the bulging, migrated portion of the nucleus back through the fissures toward the center of the disc and away from the pain-sensitive structures. Some may dispute the physiology, but experience has shown that more than any other self-care intervention repeated back bends and neck retraction movements generate the greatest immediate and long-lasting relief when applied correctly. In short, they offset the deleterious effects of the flexion-biased lifestyle.

Extension Exercises for Cervical Discogenic Conditions

For neck, midscapular, or arm symptoms that fit the derangement syndrome description, start with neck retraction movements. The key is to be consistent with the neck movements. Glide your neck back as shown, pausing at the end point to place pressure on but not cause pain to the neck or upper back. The general guideline is 10 to 12 repetitions every two or three hours, especially after a long period of sitting or desk work. Begin with the doorway stretch and neck retraction. After a successful start in which you feel no lasting increase of midscapular or arm symptoms, progress to the next series.

Seated or Standing

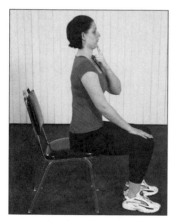

Neck Retraction

Sit on the edge of a chair or stand. Glide your head back on your neck, keeping the chin level to the floor. Avoid looking up or down. It may be helpful to use your finger as a guide, pushing on the chin. Feel pressure or movement where the neck meets the torso, the cervicaothoracic junction. Do 10 to 12 repetitions every two to three hours.

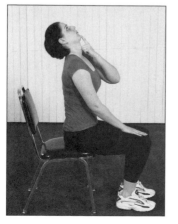

Neck Retraction With Extension

The starting position is the same as for the neck retraction exercise. Sit on the edge of a chair or stand. Glide your head back on your neck, keeping the chin level to the floor. When your head is all the way back, look up toward the ceiling. Be careful to move at the junction of the neck and upper back, not only the neck. Feel pressure and movement where the neck meets the upper torso, not just at the neck. Keep the retracted position as you look up. This exercise is an excellent way to resolve neck discogenic issues and gain much needed mobility of the upper trunk. Do 10 to 12 repetitions every two to three hours.

Extension Exercises for Lumbar Discogenic Conditions

For lower back, buttock, or leg symptoms that fit the derangement syndrome description, start with prone extension exercises. Move through the following series of activities, described in order, progressing from one to the other as long as no discomfort is produced farther down your arm or leg.

The key is to be consistent with the extension activities. The general guideline is 10 to 12 repetitions of one of the movements every two or three hours, especially after a long commute, a period of sitting, or forward-bending work.

If you are in acute pain, doing the stabilization exercises initially is not necessary. Use the neck and lower back extension activities for a week or two before beginning the stabilization program. This progression will help protect against aggravating the disc while straining during the exercises.

If you've had discomfort for more than three months, begin the stabilization activities a day or two after commencing the neck and back movements. As always, none of the activities should produce any lasting increase of symptoms.

For both neck and lower back symptoms, you may notice an increase of symptoms closer to your spine following the exercises. This is a good sign of progress as long as the symptoms in your arm or leg are diminishing. Yes, a decrease of arm and leg symptoms is good in spite of an increase in shoulder blade or buttock pain. From there, the shoulder blade or buttock pain should subside, although your neck or low back discomfort may increase. As symptoms subside away from your arm or leg, you may have an increase of localized discomfort closer to the trunk. This result is a sign of progress. The clinical term is centralization. The greater the distance your symptoms are from your spine, the longer the recuperation period is. Be patient and look for signs of centralization, which is an indication that you are on the right track.

Prone

Prone on Elbows

Lie propped up on your elbows and allow your back to sag. Maintain this position for two to three minutes. If you have acute symptoms, perform this exercise several times a day. If you have chronic symptoms, perform the exercise periodically.

Prone Press-Ups

Lie on your belly (*a*). Using your arms only, press yourself up into a back bend (*b*). The back should remain at rest; the upper arms do all the work. Do 10 to 12 repetitions at a time. If you have acute symptoms, perform the exercise several times a day. If your symptoms are chronic, perform the exercise periodically. Move the hands farther away or closer to you to achieve a different feel. Use the hand placement that feels best.

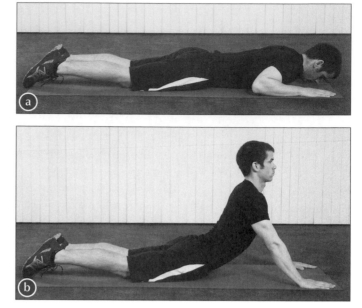

Standing

Standing Back Bend

Stand with your hands on your hips (*a*). Bend back (*b*). Do not bend the knees. You don't need to move far. For a more specific stretch, move your hands farther behind you, placing the thumbs at the top of the tailbone to act as a fulcrum to pivot off as you bend back. In this way you can isolate the back bend at the exact level where you feel the source of the discomfort. For acute symptoms do 10 to 12 repetitions every few hours. For more chronic complaints try to do the exercise several times a day, especially after longer bouts of sitting.

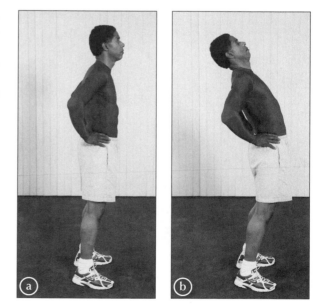

Evaluate Your Routine

Jim is a mental health clinician who travels a lot. He developed a curvature in his back and reported that his lower back pain was worsening. The clinical examination confirmed what was provoking his symptoms, but what brought it on was not readily apparent. After we discussed his exercise routine, the culprit became painfully clear. He had used the same exercise regimen for many years, but what was once helpful had become hurtful. What Jim began years ago to stay in shape had become irritating to the disc and was provoking his symptoms.

His condition responded quickly with the addition of some simple back bends. The real lasting benefit, however, came from a complete revision of his exercise program. The revision removed the activities that put more pressure on the disc and replaced them with some of the exercises described in this chapter. Often the best remedy is to stop the aggravating element, which is why body mechanics and office ergonomics are covered in chapters 6 and 7, respectively.

Jim's story illustrates the importance of analyzing your routine. What once was helpful may need a little updating. Any good trainer or therapist can help you with this.

Remember to pay attention to the voices of your symptoms. If a dull neck ache or backache gradually turns into a pain down your arm or leg or numbness develops, your condition may have changed to a more serious problem. In these cases additional medical intervention is appropriate. Remember that an accurate diagnosis is needed to develop an accurate treatment plan.

Extension Exercises for Thoracic Compression Fractures

The upper back mobility stretch described on page 63 is appropriate to treat thoracic compression fractures, as are the chest-out postural exercises described on page 57 Avoid bending forward, especially when lifting. Pay close attention to body mechanics as described in chapter 5 to minimize lumbar flexion strain. Be sure to focus on the golfer's lift technique also described in chapter 6.

Flexion-Biased Exercises for Lumbar Spondylolisthesis

The stabilization series of exercises described earlier in the chapter works great for lumbar spondylolisthesis. Avoiding prone leg lifts is often beneficial because bending back the lower spine can worsen the discomfort. Seated forward bending provides a nice stretch for relief as do stretches for the front of the hip.

BALANCE ACTIVITIES

Although balance activities don't fit the definition of exercise in the strength-building world, balance training offers many benefits for the short time needed to practice it. Balance can be improved with practice. All of us can use the benefits of balance training to complement a well-rounded exercise regimen. Begin by performing the activities with your eyes open. Then, after you're successful, try them with your eyes closed. Studies show that your risk of falling is greater when you cannot maintain a single-leg stance position for at least five seconds. Improving your ability to stand on one leg will reduce your risk of falling.

Standing

Single-Leg Stance

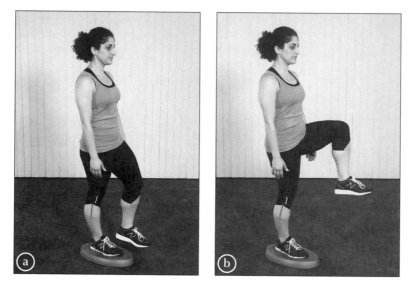

Stand on an unstable surface such as a soft pad. If you need extra support to help your balance, perform this exercise near a wall or sturdy object that you can use for support. Stand on one leg, keeping the knee of the standing leg slightly unlocked (a). Hold the lifted leg with the knee up toward your chest (b). Keep your eyes open for an easier activity or close your eyes for a harder one. Maintain the single-leg stance as long as you can, up to 20 seconds. Switch legs. Try several repetitions on each side.

GYM CONSIDERATIONS

If you choose to go to a gym, you need to be aware of which common gym activities tend to aggravate various spinal conditions. These generalizations do not always apply, but they warrant consideration.

Those with a diagnosis of neck discogenic pain should avoid the seated overhead press and lateral raise. Watch your head position if you choose to use a regular or stationary bike because this activity often produces symptoms. Sit up tall and look forward instead of slumping and looking at the ground.

Those with a diagnosis of lumbar discogenic pain should avoid the seated leg press, seated overhead press, and seated biceps curl. These exercises often aggravate symptoms. If you feel better over time, do them cautiously.

Those with spondylolisthesis diagnoses should avoid the behind-the-back pull-down, standing military press, standing biceps curl, and trunk rotation. Avoid trunk extensions. It is best to complete any standing exercise with the feet slightly staggered and avoid side-by-side positioning. Be sure to engage your bracing muscles and proceed slowly.

Those with a diagnosis of cervical stenosis should avoid the overhead press and be cautious regarding the chest press. Those with lumbar stenosis should be wary of the same set of activities noted for spondylolisthesis because they can cause pressure on the spinal cord, leading to much greater concerns.

Those with arm and leg symptoms described as deep, burning, or aching should be careful when stretching. In acute situations, pulling on an already irritated nerve root is unwise. For the arm, keep the hand on your abdomen when you stretch. For the leg, be sure to keep your knee bent and proceed conservatively, assessing how you feel after completing a stretch.

ISOMETRICS

In addition to the trunk stabilization programs, isometric exercises can be a useful part of your home trunk care program. By definition, an isometric contraction is one in which no movement about the joint axis takes place. In practical terms, you simply push or pull against a nonmoveable resistance to gain the advantage of contracting a muscle without creating shear, torsion, and loading forces across a joint. This activity promotes strengthening without the associated irritation of the spinal structures.

Isometric exercises are useful because they address two specific issues common to gym-based and other activity-based programs. Often well-intended exercise routines are put on hold because they cause pain and demand a lot of time. The following exercises minimize the likelihood of pain common to those who start new gym programs. They also make efficient use of time because they can be done at home without any equipment in less than 20 minutes.

The concept is based on using the advantage of time. Gym-based programs commonly use a 10 to 12 repetition set, and each repetition takes generally one second to do. At a weight of 50 pounds (23 kg), one set would accomplish generally 500 units of work ($50 \times 10 \times 1$). In the isometric program, the resistance is dramatically reduced, minimizing the likelihood of tissue injury. For example, assume a 20-pound (9 kg) force and no more than 5 repetitions. The duration of the contraction is significantly longer at 20 seconds or more. Computing the general level of work in this case provides us with 2,000 units of work (20 × 5 × 20) for one set. Although the resistance was lower and the number of repetitions was reduced by half, the isometric set created more overall work demand on the muscles due to the longer duration of the contraction.

Isometric exercises are safe for those with aching joints and convenient because no equipment is necessary. The American Rheumatology Association recommends isometric exercises to help reverse osteoporosis and treat osteoarthritis. The American Neurological Association reports that isometric exercises, when done correctly, increase production of brain cells. Here are a few isometric exercises to add to your workout program.

Myth

I HAVE ARTHRITIS SO I SHOULDN'T EXERCISE

On the contrary, the fact you have arthritis makes it more important to exercise. The key is to do a program that helps you make progress.

An arthritic joint that becomes painful inhibits the muscles that cross that joint, leading to further pain. As the condition worsens, you begin to compensate in the way that you walk, reach forward, or bend and twist. Eventually, arthritis creates compensations in the neck and lower back that worsen discomfort in those areas.

Perhaps the best way to begin an exercise routine if you have painful, arthritic joints is with isometrics. By definition, isometrics refers to a muscle contraction during which no movement about the joint takes place, such as pushing against a wall. As you press against the wall, the muscles in your arm contract, but no motion takes place. In addition, there is no external resistance. You generate all the force. You can work as hard or as gently as your symptoms allow. Isometrics allow you to work the muscles without moving the painful joint.

For conditions relating to the spine, clinicians often use trunk stabilization exercises (see page 45). These exercises force you to activate your trunk muscles without eliciting spinal discomfort. Trunk isometrics form the basis of our self-help intervention program. The nice thing about isometrics is that you don't have to go to a gym or have access to any equipment to do them. All you need is will power and the desire to get better.

Upper Extremities

Chest Press and Pull

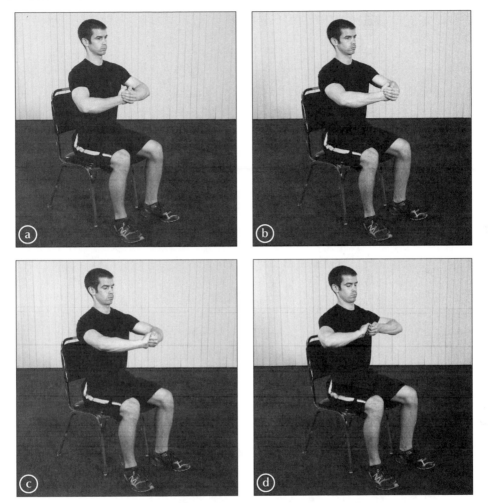

Press your hands together as if trying to smash one hand into the other (a). Hold for five counts. Then, while maintaining the pressure, move your hands slightly away from you for five counts (b). Hold this new position for five counts and repeat. When your arms are completely in front of you, interlock your fingers and try to pull your shoulder blades together (c). Hold for five counts. Then, while maintaining the pressure, move your hands closer to you for five counts (d). Hold the new position for five counts and repeat. Do five repetitions in each direction.

Biceps and Triceps

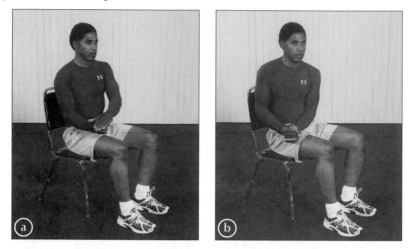

Sit or stand. Place an open hand over the closed fist of the other hand (a). Resist bending your elbow (elbow flexion) by applying gentle pressure from the open palm hand down onto the fist. Slowly allow the elbow to bend, moving up for five counts. When the elbow is fully bent, move the top hand beneath the closed fist (b) to repeat in the other direction, forcing the arm back down for five counts while applying resistance with the open hand. Stop and hold at several points along the way. Do five repetitions in each direction for each side.

Lower Extremities

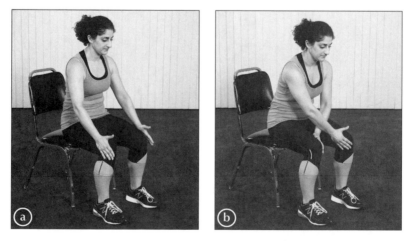

Hip In and Out

Begin in a seated position. Use your hands to apply pressure against the outer knees (a). Use your arms to resist the pressure of your knees pushing out for a full five-second count. Switch your hands to the inner knees (b) and apply resistance as you try to bring your knees together for a five-second count. Repeat, resisting the movement of the knees outward and then inward, each taking five counts. Stop and hold at several points along the way. Do five repetitions in each direction.

Partial Squat and Heel Raise

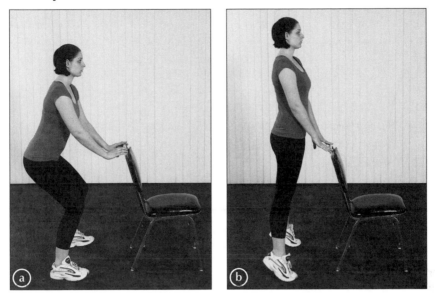

Assume a partial squat position with feet shoulder-width apart, toes forward, and hips back as if you are sitting down (a). Rest your hands on your hips or hold onto a sturdy object for balance. Lower yourself for five counts and then return to standing in five counts. When you are fully upright, slowly rise onto your toes for five counts (b). Slowly lower yourself back to the starting position for five counts and repeat the sequence. Do five repetitions.

STEPS TO SELF-CARE

This chapter will not teach you a complete therapy program or provide a specific personal training routine. Too many variables are at play—symptoms, diagnoses, lifestyle factors, individual skill level—to design a routine that is safe for all readers. We do provide safe self-help activities as a starting point to ease your back and neck pain. The exercises and stretches described should not elicit a lasting increase in discomfort. If you find yourself getting worse, it doesn't mean that you're doing the wrong program. It may mean that you are doing an exercise the wrong way or that an exercise is not right for you. Go slowly and pay attention to how you feel with each exercise. Rather than stop altogether, simply take one stretch or exercise out of the mix and see how you do. Chances are that only one exercise out of the five or six that you are doing is causing a problem. Try to identify that one and stick with the others. In the long run, you'll be glad you did.

Studies show that many types of exercise and stretching programs are helpful. There is no one right way. Often it's not the specifics of what you do, but rather that you are doing something. You have a lot to say in the outcome of your spinal discomfort, but it does take effort. There is no magic pill. By increasing flexibility, improving strength, and developing cardiovascular fitness, you are taking a positive step toward feeling better.

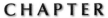

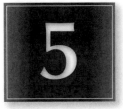

Making Lifestyle Choices to Ease Pain

Most health care practitioners agree that lifestyle influences have a significant role in the onset or alleviation of spinal pain. Incorporating lifestyle changes can have a significant and lasting effect on reducing, eliminating, and preventing recurrent spinal discomfort.

In this chapter, we address five specific lifestyle factors—fitness level, diet and nutrition, sleep, smoking, and stress—and show you how they affect spinal pain. We provide simple self-help guidelines for each and show you how small changes can have a large and lasting effect. That you can control these factors makes your chances of success all the better.

"Wait a minute," you say, "What about age? I'm not getting any younger, and my spinal pain is getting worse." Spinal pain and age are connected to some degree. Several conditions such as spinal stenosis and spondylosis do become more frequent as we age. But the point of this chapter is to discuss the lifestyle choices that we can control, those that undoubtedly affect the onset of or the severity of spinal pain. Aging is not something that we can control. We all age at exactly the same rate, one day at a time. So although aging does lead to a gradual loss of flexibility, strength, and the ability to recuperate, the five lifestyle factors that we can control are the concern of this chapter. If you manage these five factors appropriately, you can significantly diminish spinal pain or prevent it from occurring.

THE SCIENCE OF HEALTH

Before we begin, we need to examine a bit of science to help us understand why these lifestyle factors can benefit or hinder your progress. A basic understanding of cellular biology, tissue strength, and oxygen transport will illuminate why the body reacts as it does to these specific lifestyle choices.

Let's begin with cellular biology. Picture a classic car that is kept covered in the garage. As long as the car is kept covered and stored safely in the garage, it poses no concern. If you want to take it for a spin, you need only one thing—fuel for the engine. Without fuel, the car is useless. It will look good regardless, but if you want to use it, you've got to gas it up. After the car is filled up, the quality and efficiency of the engine becomes the next key factor in how that car will perform. Are all the cylinders working properly? Is the timing correct? Is the engine putting out the maximal horsepower that it is capable of? Does the engine have enough size and stamina to move the car through town, up a mountainside, across the country?

The car analogy is relevant to your body because similar factors are at play on a cellular level. Your cells also need fuel to perform properly. Whereas gasoline makes the car engine function, oxygen is the required fuel to make the cell motor work. Without enough gas, the shiny classic sitting in the garage is not going to get you around town or even down the block. Similarly, without enough oxygen, the cells of your body cannot keep you healthy and pain free for a week, month, or year.

Oxygen is to the cell as gas is to the car. Without oxygen, the cell won't function properly. The engine of the cell is the mitochondria. Mitochondria, the cell's energy-producing unit, are numerous within each cell. They transform fuel into energy and ultimately make the cell do what it is intended to do. Mitochondria are more numerous and larger in size when the cell gets more oxygen, but they shrivel in number and size when oxygen transport to the cell diminishes. When the mitochondria are plentiful and well fueled, the cell is more resilient and tolerant to daily stress and strain.

The key factor to cellular health is the presence and delivery of oxygen to the cell. Factors that impede the ability of the vascular system to deliver oxygen reduce the ability of the cell to tolerate day-to-day strain. Factors that improve the transport of oxygen to the cell improve cellular resiliency. With cellular resiliency comes greater tissue strength.

When asked to define strength, many say that it is the ability to lift something, produce a force, or exert effort. All are true, but none correct in the context of tissue strength. In this regard, compare tissue wrapping paper to a piece of cardboard, cotton fabric to a burlap bag, or balsa wood to oak. Which is stronger? Which can tolerate repeated stresses, and which is better able to withstand day-to-day wear and tear? If a cup of water is placed on a wet piece of tissue paper, would it keep the cup from falling through as well as a wet piece of cardboard would? Would you feel as secure standing on a ladder made of balsa wood as you would on one made of oak? The analogy of stronger applies to cells as well. Those with superior levels of oxygen and energy production demonstrate greater resiliency to the daily wear and tear that tend to break us down. These stronger cells will be more resistant to breakdown and the subsequent symptoms. Oxygen transport is the key.

Common to each of the five lifestyle factors discussed in this chapter is the effect that each has on the delivery of oxygen and nutrients to the cells. By enhancing your fitness, improving your nutrition, promoting restful sleep, controlling stress, and avoiding smoking, you increase blood flow throughout your body, including the joints, bones, muscles, and connective tissues of the back and neck. Also important is the benefit of removing built-up toxins and metabolic wastes from the tissues. The perfusion of oxygen-rich blood to the cells is an important factor in maintaining cellular health and recuperative capacity. If your cells are deprived of the necessary fuels for too long, you will experience symptoms such as pain, aching, stiffness, swelling, or ongoing tightness, among others. As you manage these lifestyle factors in a positive way, the tissues become more resilient to the stresses and strains that you encounter every day. You will achieve an overall benefit to your spinal health.

LIFESTYLE FACTOR 1: FITNESS LEVEL

You may be thinking, "Here it comes, another doctor telling me I have to go to the gym five days a week, pump some iron, run a 10K, and be as flexible as a gymnast." Yes, fitness is important, but achieving it does not require as much time and work as you might think. The health care community agrees that overall fitness level directly influences the success of treatment for spinal pain. The North American Spine Society advocates fitness to enhance the health of your spine, as does nearly every other health care credentialing body. Based on our experience, those who are more fit get better faster and more routinely. Those who become more fit are able to recover better than they did before.

Getting in shape does not require a major time commitment or drain all your energy. To begin, we should first define what we mean by fitness level and then relate it to specific activities for your spine.

For general fitness (see table 5.1), the American College of Sports Medicine (ACSM) and the American Heart Association recommend 30 minutes a day, 5 days a week, of moderately intense cardiovascular training or 20 minutes of cardiovascular training combined with approximately 20 minutes of strength training 3 days a week. For those over 65, they advocate adding a balance activity to the routine. When training at moderate intensity, you should still be able to carry on a conversation.

Table 5.1 General Fitness Guidelines

	Cardiovascular exercise	Strength training	Flexibility	Balance
Younger than 65 years old	30 minutes a day, 5 days a week, or 20 minutes a day, 3 days a week when combined with strength training	8 to 10 exercises at 8 to 12 repetitions per set	Movement-based warm-up for 5 to 10 minutes before workout Static stretches for 10 to 15 minutes after workout	Not specifically recommended
65 years old and older	30 minutes a day, 5 days a week, or 20 minutes a day, 5 days a week, when combined with strength training	8 to 10 exercises at 10 to 15 repetitions per set	Movement-based warm-up for 5 to 10 minutes before workout Static stretches for 10 to 15 minutes after workout	Recommended

EXERCISING AT HOME WILL HELP MY NECK OR BACK

This statement may or may not be true, depending on what exercise you are doing. Generally, the more fit you are, the more likely you are to minimize or eliminate your spinal discomfort. That said, you can aggravate your condition in the process of getting or staying in shape. Not all fitness activities are the same.

Exercise programs can take many forms, from traditional weightlifting to jogging and biking, from sports such as basketball and golf to yoga, Pilates, and tai chi. Each has merit for improving your overall health. Some, however, may be counterproductive, worsening your spinal discomfort.

Jim is a young, strong construction worker who has chronic lower back pain. He can't figure out why his lower back aches. Jim likes to use a leg press machine at the gym. These machines are trouble for those with discogenic problems. After Jim stopped that one activity, his symptoms began to resolve.

Jack is an overweight patient who is trying to get back in shape. He walked mile after mile on his treadmill, only to stop after several months because of severe and increasing leg pain. The walking created so much irritation to his already compressed lower back that the nerve roots became swollen and irritated, hindering rather than helping his progress.

Jane is a middle-aged computer user who has poor posture and unrelenting shoulder pain. She not only worked at a computer all day and often at home at night but also liked to do push-ups, which irritated the problem. Push-ups often irritate an overworked rotator cuff tendon. Temporarily changing her activities enabled Jane to stay active as her shoulders healed.

Ask yourself whether you generally have more spinal discomfort or feel worse the morning after a workout. If so, chances are that your exercise program is contributing to your neck or back issue. Try implementing some of the activities in the book for a while and see how you feel. Often a little foundation building allows you to return to all or part of your prior exercise regime and feel much better for doing it.

Cardiovascular Training

Cardiovascular conditioning includes many forms of activity. Commonly used gym equipment includes stationary bikes, treadmills, elliptical trainers, and arm ergometers or arm bikes. You may include any activity that you find enjoyable and does not seem to worsen your pain. Swimming is an excellent form of exercise for those with spinal pain because of the buoyancy properties of water. Those with extension sensitive conditions such as stenosis, spondylosis, or spondylolisthesis may find flexion-based activities such as biking, rowing, or using a seated ergometer more tolerable, whereas those with flexion-sensitive conditions such as disc prolapse, compression fractures, or postural discomfort may find extension-biased activities such as walking, using an elliptical machine, or swimming especially useful.

Regardless of the type of cardiovascular conditioning that you choose, cardiovascular training promotes both oxygen transport (picking up oxygen from the lungs) and oxygen delivery (dropping off the oxygen molecule to the tissues). The goal is to get your heart rate in the target zone (see figure 5.1) for 20 to 30 consecutive minutes. To find your target zone, use this formula:

$$(220 - age) \times 0.60 \text{ to } 0.85 / 4 = \text{pulse count per 15 seconds}$$

For example, to achieve a cardiovascular benefit, a 45-year-old would strive for a pulse rate during exercise of 26 to 37 beats per 15 seconds:

$$220 - 45 = 175$$
$$175 \times 0.60 = 105$$
$$105 / 4 = 26.25 \text{ (round down to 26)}$$
$$175 \times 0.85 = 148.75 \text{ (round up to 149)}$$
$$149 / 4 = 37.25 \text{ (round down to 37)}$$

Therefore, the 45-year-old would have to work hard enough to get his heart rate above 105 beats per minute but to remain safe not above 149 beats per minute.

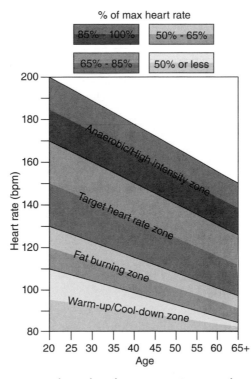

Figure 5.1   Heart rate zones based on beats per minute and age.

The easiest place to take your pulse is the inside of your wrist just above the fold. Another easy access site is under the jawbone along the side of your neck just lateral to the Adam's apple.

Cardiovascular conditioning also promotes the release of endorphins, your body's natural pain killers. Endorphins work to moderate your perception of pain and are released after bouts of cardiovascular activity. This effect causes the runner's high, the ability of some athletes to carry on in spite of injury or illness. These natural opiates are important because they provide a good feeling that results from the effort you put in at the gym or at home. They provide a sense of well-being after a day of particularly hard work or exercise. Maintaining a level of endorphins in your blood stream can help diminish the sensation of pain and lessen the anxiety that goes along with it. Cardiovascular conditioning is a great way to naturally ease anxiety and the sensation of pain.

Strength Training

Strength training is necessary for a well-rounded level of fitness. Among the many forms of muscle strength training are weightlifting, Pilates, yoga, and isometrics. In most cases, regardless of the form of strength training used, as long as the parameters are correct and the specific activity that you choose does not elicit a lasting increase in pain, you will experience some gain in muscle strength. By gaining muscle strength, you are on your way toward combating spinal pain.

A properly developed strength program incorporates several factors. First, consider your starting level of fitness. If you're a novice, you'll make faster progress if you start slowly. Take your time and spend the first 6 to 10 weeks learning how to work out. The three primary reasons that a fitness program fails and you do not achieve your fitness goals are a lack of time, not having any fun, and getting injured. You can address the last two simply by finding activities that you like and incorporating them into your daily regimen slowly and methodically. If you've been on a strengthening or fitness program recently, you may resume a bit more quickly but remember that if it's no fun and you get hurt, you won't stick with it. Go slowly and find weight-training activities that you enjoy.

Second, assess your current ability and stay within your limits. For a weightlifting program, use the repetition maximum (RM) scale as a guide to workout intensity. Generally, a reasonable starting point is a bout of exercise, called a set, of 15 to 20 repetitions. You should be able to lift the weight 15 to 20 times without a change in technique or posture but not more than that before fatigue. If you can lift a weight more than 20 times, the weight is too light. If you cannot lift the weight 15 times, it is too heavy. When starting a gym weight-training program, work at 15 to 20 RM loads for one set of each exercise. Before adding weight, add a second set. Adjust your program to meet your specific training goals but keep the RM scale in mind and use a 6- to 10-week learning period to avoid injury. After you are comfortable, add weight until you can do at least 12 repetitions but not more than 15. For muscle hypertrophy and enhanced strength, add weight until you can do at least 10 repetitions but no more than 12. This 10- to 12-repetition range will provide a level of safety and enhance strength building. Remember that a weight-training program should not cause spinal discomfort, should be fun, and should not impose a large time drain on your day.

A final consideration in beginning a strength-training program is the type of activity that you'll do. Although walking, dancing, golf, and yard work are forms of exercise, none offer the benefits of true strengthening that your spine needs to stay healthy and symptom free. Loading, or placing added strain on your muscles and bones, provides the benefits of a strengthening program. You need the added load that weight training, yoga, and Pilates offer to stimulate your body to enlarge your muscles, strengthen your bones, and release endorphins.

For those interested in firming and toning hard-to-get areas, maintain the cardiovascular conditioning concepts addressed earlier and add 20 to 30 minutes of weight training at loads of 15 to 20 RM. Working in a circuit—doing one set of each exercise followed by a second set of each exercise—will provide the benefit of cardiovascular training while you condition and tone your muscles. Remember that even at a load of 10 to 12 RM, no lasting discomfort or short-term tendon or joint pain should occur after the exercise session. Muscle soreness is acceptable, but tendon and joint pain is not. If you are sore and experience lasting stiffness, stop the weight training and consult your physical therapist or physician. If you choose activities that incorporate body weight as the resistance, such as Pilates or yoga, the same general guidelines apply. These programs offer the advantage that many of the activities are done in gravity-minimized positions. You can adjust the loading on your spine more closely, taking into account pain and other limiting issues. No form of exercise is perfect; each offers merit where some other does not. By balancing your activities over the course of a year, referred to as periodizing the program, you allow your body to benefit from different activities while minimizing the likelihood of musculoskeletal pain and strain common with overuse and overloading.

Contrary to some beliefs, weight training is crucial to maintaining a healthy spine. To increase functional ability, the body must be exposed to greater workloads than normally encountered during typical day-to-day tasks. Because walking, dancing, golf, housework, and the like do not offer greater loads than normally encountered during the course of a day, in and of themselves they cannot be considered strength-gaining

Consider Isometrics

For those unable to make it to a gym, isometric exercises provide a great way to accomplish strength-training goals. Isometric exercise, muscle contraction in which no joint movement takes place, aides in promoting circulatory function while working to strengthen muscles. Isometrics are a great choice for strengthening and increasing bone density, especially in postmenopausal women. Like everything else, isometrics have limitations. But to accomplish the goals of helping to maintain circulatory, neuromuscular, and muscle performance, isometrics are an excellent choice. For more on isometrics, see chapter 4.

activities. Only by placing an added load on the muscles, joints, and spine can an activity offer the benefits of strengthening. Incorporating a 20- to 30-minute strengthening component three days a week, beginning at 15 to 20 RM and slowly progressing to 10 to 12 RM, will enable you to begin promoting the muscle strength and capacity necessary to support your spine.

Resistance training promotes circulatory function and oxygen delivery to the cell's engine by maintaining an efficient vascular system. Additionally, the pumping action of the muscles during the workout helps to move fluids along the venous system back toward the heart for completion of the circulatory cycle.

Flexibility

Cardiovascular conditioning and strength training are important components of a fitness program. One often overlooked aspect of fitness is flexibility. Across all ages, flexibility is of particular importance for general health and especially for the spine. Just as we may try to stretch a dollar or perhaps occasionally stretch the truth, we should be mindful of the need to stretch the muscles and supporting myofascia, the sinews that surround the spine and hold us together.

Stretching may be overlooked because it offers no outwardly obvious benefit. Men typically lift weights in an effort to get a big chest or ripped arm and leg muscles, or they may play weekend sports in an attempt to stay young. Women seem to prefer activities that slim their waistlines while toning the muscles. They often choose group activities such as yoga, Pilates, or aerobic classes and tend to avoid the bulk-building activities of the men. Often the time it takes to stretch is viewed as cool-down time, an afterthought, left for the last few minutes of a workout session before the ride home or a quick shower. Yet clinical experience reveals that stretching is the most important part of the program for most people dealing with spinal pain and dysfunction. Degenerative conditions of the spine, stenosis, radiculopathy, overuse and muscle tension issues, athletics-related injuries, adaptive shortening, and many other types of conditions respond well to stretching.

The benefits of stretching are many. Stretching promotes a larger range of motion, reduces muscle tension, enhances circulation, and improves oxygen delivery to the tissues by reducing the mechanical constriction of the vessels from the surrounding connective tissue and muscle tissue tension. The effect is similar to what happens if you stand on the middle of your garden hose and then step off. Clearly, the amount of water flowing out the end increases after you take your foot off the hose. By reducing tissue tension, you improve circulation.

Developing a stretching program needn't be difficult, although to do it correctly you need to invest some time and perhaps seek the guidance of a qualified professional. Some trained clinicians advocate stretching tight muscles by holding the stretch for 10 seconds and completing three repetitions or so, or holding for 30 seconds before moving to the next stretch, or something of the sort. Although the literature does not specifically state the right amount of time to hold a stretch or recommend a specific frequency for performing stretches, empirically we know that a few bouts of 10-second holds are far too short to gain actual length of short-ened myofascia or diminish active muscle tone. Practically, holding a stretch for at least 60 seconds a minimum of two times for each stretch offers some tissue tension relief and a temporary gain of movement ease. Although not validated scientifically, holding the stretch for a minimum of 60 seconds several times is a good starting point. Those with true muscular shortening will need to progress to holding the stretch for several minutes and repeating two or three times as a final ending point. Fortunately, developing a stretching program is not especially difficult and requires less apparatus and time than a gym or swimming workout.

The skeletal muscles that move your body can be categorized into two main groups. Postural muscles cross more than one joint and are prone to shortness. Phasic, or movement-oriented, muscles cross just one joint and are prone to weak-ness. Most often, flexibility loss follows a general pattern, making it easy to predict which areas and muscles to stretch. Your health care provider should be able to identify the pattern and prescribe the proper stretches in a straightforward manner. (We provide examples and suggestions of what to do in chapter 4.) When done correctly, stretching nearly always has a beneficial effect on the target area. At all times, stretching should feel good. It should never feel noxious or gritty. Usually, stretching is a necessary and beneficial component of a therapeutic program. By targeting the multijoint postural muscles in the area needing greater flexibility, you can achieve a symptomatic and functional benefit in a short time. But when stretching is done wrong or the wrong stretches are used, stretching likely is going to be a source of irritation, compounding the original problem.

Many patients and clinicians believe that stretching the hamstrings, the group of muscles along the back of the upper thigh, is important to ease lower back pain. In some cases, hamstring stretches are useful because the hamstrings are multijoint muscles that tend to become short. Hamstring flexibility is necessary for resolving some low back pain, and often poor hamstring flexibility is a contributing cause. But remember the story of Donna from chapter 4 (page 63). In her case, even though the hamstrings fit the pattern of being tight, stretching them when she was in acute pain was a recipe for disaster. When asked why Donna had done that particular series of stretches, her therapist replied that it was because Donna had tight hamstrings. Without proper assessment, an irritated nerve or nerve root will commonly present as a tight muscle. By stretching that hamstring, Donna's therapist further irritated an already irritated nerve root, quickly exacerbating the leg pain.

Balance

Balance training is an important part of any physical fitness routine, especially for those 65 and older. Each year, more than one-third of those 65 and over fall, making falls the leading cause of deaths and most common cause of nonfatal injury in older adults. The American Physical Therapy Association provides materials on the pre-vention of falls. In it, they note four main aspects to minimize the risk of falling: physical conditioning, yearly vision examinations, home safety assessment, and a medication review with a doctor.

You can perform several self-checks to assess your risk of falling. The easiest is to count the number of medications that you take daily. Taking more than three medications per day has been shown to cause a significant increase in the risk of falling. Narcotics such as vicodan, oxycontin, and methadone are particularly dangerous, especially when taken in combination with tranquilizers, muscle relaxers, or sleep medications. Another self-check is to assess how far you can reach forward. Stand with your feet shoulder-width apart and your arm held out in front of you and then measure how far you can reach forward. If the total distance is 10 inches (25 cm) or more, your risk of falling is small. If it is less than 6 inches (15 cm), you are four times more likely to fall, and if it is less than 4 inches (10 cm), you are six times more likely to fall. A final simple self-check is the single-limb stance test. Studies show that if you are able to stand on one leg without any other support or contact for five seconds or longer, you are less likely to fall than someone who cannot stand on one leg for at least five seconds.

Balance activities are effective and simple and do not require additional equipment. Because balance is a skill, you can improve it by practicing it. Place your feet side by side and reach forward, keeping 10 inches (25 cm) or more as your goal. Stand on one leg for as long as you can or stand in a heel-to-toe position while you reach, bend, or twist. As long as you are safe and have objects nearby for support if you need it, progress in these activities by trying them with your eyes open and then closed. For some good balance exercises, see chapter 4 (page 72).

LIFESTYLE FACTOR 2: DIET AND NUTRITION

The importance of maintaining a healthy diet is something that we're all aware of, but it seems hard for many of us to do. Public health officials agree that the fattening of the American population is a problem that includes many factors, related not only to the availability of fast food and junk food but also to lifestyle, academic, family, and social pressures. The added girth of the American population has put a strain on the overall health of our nation. Consider these facts:

- In 1960 the average American male weighed 166 pounds (75 kg). Forty years later he weighed 191 pounds (86 kg). In 1960 the average American female weighed 140 pounds (64 kg). Forty years later she weighed 164 pounds (74 kg).

- In 1985 eight states reported adult obesity rates greater than 10 percent. By 1994 all states had rates greater than 10 percent and 16 states had rates above 15 percent. By 2004 all but seven states were above 20 percent and nine states were above 25 percent. In 2007 four states were above 30 percent. By the end of 2010 the obesity rate across the United States had reached 31 percent.

- In the mid-1970s childhood and adolescent obesity rates were 4 percent and 6 percent, respectively. By 2008 they had leveled at 19 percent and 17 percent, respectively.

- The average American child today eats 780 calories more per day than he or she did in 1967, mostly because of the high-fructose corn syrup in foods and drinks. In 1967 only 3,000 tons of high-fructose corn syrup were produced;

today over 6,000,000 tons are made. Some reports note a one in three likeli-hood that those born in 2000 or later will develop type 2 diabetes, leading to a lifespan decrease of 17 to 27 years.

- As reported in the *San Francisco Chronicle* in June 2009, Illinois remained one of only two states that required mandatory physical education participation for students of all school ages. (Massachusetts was recently added.) Even so, as of 2007, Illinois was one of the states with adult obesity rates above 25 percent.

- In 2000 the U.S. surgeon general designated obesity as a national epidemic, reaching across all ethnic and economic groups. A war on fat was declared. By 2007 the obesity rate had increased another 7 percent. More than 30 percent of adults (more than 60 million people) were considered overweight or obese (about 30 pounds [14 kg] or more overweight).

- In 1980 an average box of popcorn contained 270 calories. Today it's 630 calo-ries. In 1980 an average turkey sandwich had 320 calories. Today's supersized, overdone turkey sandwich has 820 calories or more.

Studies show that the odds of having an obese child increase considerably when one or more of the adults at home are obese or if the adults themselves were obese as children. The cycle of obesity perpetuates itself, and our health care system is bearing the burden. Costs associated with diabetes and metabolic and cardiac con-ditions are skyrocketing. In fact, many researchers report that in the 21st century we're in danger of reversing the steady increase in average lifespan made in the past 100 years simply because we're eating too much and moving too little. To some degree the increasing prevalence of spinal pain is a result of that weight gain and sedentary lifestyle.

The Problem of Overweight

In a purely mechanical sense, added weight, especially in the abdominal area, places more strain on the musculature and noncontractile elements of the spine. But we are interested in the burgeoning obesity rates for more than just the mechanical factors that affect the spine. The point of this section is not to lament the issue of weight gain itself, but to relate weight gain to spinal pain through a variety of repercussive factors. Like most everything (excluding death and taxes), there are exceptions to the rule. We all know overweight people who have no specific spinal discomfort and people who are thin but have plenty of neck and lower back discomfort. By and large, however, you are more prone to experience spinal pain if you carry excessive weight. If we revert to our initial hypothesis—all things being equal, the greater your level of fitness, the lesser the likelihood of spinal pain—being obese or overweight lessens your level of fitness in every regard. You will exercise less, eat more poorly, get less restful sleep, and be more likely to suffer from ancillary medical problems when you are heavy. Obesity decreases growth hormones, increases levels of the stress hormone cortisol, and increases the risk of sleep apnea. We must be careful to avoid making the connection that only overweight people eat poorly or that they have spinal pain solely because they are heavy. That is obviously not the case. Being overweight itself is not necessarily the issue. Rather, the effects and results of being overweight lead to a greater likelihood of spinal discomfort.

Nutrition and Cell Health

Diet is an important lifestyle choice because it is the primary way that we replenish our fuel stores. In doing so, we provide our bodies the necessary minerals, protein, carbohydrate, and fat to use for tissue health and repair. Along with oxygen, dietary intake enables our cells to recover from one day's wear and tear and prepare for the next. Without the replenishing process the cells eventually become depleted of the necessary fuel sources. Much like your car when it is low on gas, your cells will cease to work properly. On a cellular level, without the replenishing benefits of a healthy diet the stage that follows is called exhaustion. Exhaustion is the first component of tissue breakdown, eventually leading to discomfort, pain, and, if left unchecked, disability.

This scenario will help you visualize how nutrition plays an important role in your ability to maintain a level of health and recuperate from the strain of the day. A road construction crew was working nearby, building an overpass. The day was very hot, the kind of day that could cause a person to feel drained after a walk of a just few blocks. A tall, thin, and slightly muscled worker had come out of the nearby convenience store carrying a king-sized candy bar, an oversized bag of chips, and a 64-ounce (2 L) soda. Apparently, that was his lunch. His workmate had a home-made sandwich, an apple, and a drink for lunch. Although there is no way to tell exactly what would happen, a little logic will help us predict the result. Although the worker who bought his lunch at the convenience store was thin and obviously not counting calories, he was depriving himself of the necessary benefits of proper refueling by taking on such low-quality fuel. Given the physical nature of his job, we can suspect it was simply a matter of time (or perhaps he already was there) before his cells, running on empty day after day, began to suffer the effects of fuel depletion. Tissue exhaustion and discomfort eventually follow.

Anti-Inflammatory Benefit in Chronic Pain

Diet also affects the body's response to inflammation and the duration of the inflammatory cycle. In patients with chronic pain, one consideration is the ongoing presence of an inflammatory process that heightens the transmission of pain stimulus by the nervous system. Food that contains antioxidants and other inflammatory-reducing substances can go a long way toward helping turn down the amplification of pain signals, ultimately reducing the perception of discomfort. Common anti-inflammatory foods include nuts, fish, olive oil, complex carbohydrates such as dark blue and dark green fruits and vegetables, and foods rich in omega 3 and omega 9 fatty acids.

LIFESTYLE FACTOR 3: SLEEP

A third lifestyle choice that directly affects your ability to maintain a strong and pain-free spine is your sleep habits. Sleep is the period when the body does the repairs and replenishing that you need to feel rested and rejuvenated for the following day.

Without restful sleep, the body is always in a state of catch-up. Quality sleep helps to balance your hormones, increasing the levels of serotonin and dopamine, the feel-good hormones, and decreasing the level of cortisol. Children and adolescents need nine hours, and adults need seven to eight hours of restful sleep every day.

Consider the following analogy. We each have a baggage cart that we pull daily. It's loaded with the various day-to-day strains of life—physical, emotional, and mental—each adding a burden to the baggage cart every day. During sleep, the body repairs, heals, and replenishes, effectively emptying the baggage cart to create a lighter, more manageable load for the next day. Consider what happens if the baggage cart does not fully empty at the end of the day. Gradually it becomes heavier and harder to pull. Because the cart is weighed down with leftover baggage, it becomes harder to steer. The cart may eventually overflow and create a mess to clean up.

How do you feel when you do not get enough sleep? Physically tired, mentally lethargic, sluggish? Do you have difficulty concentrating? Are you moody, short tempered, emotionally more fragile? The weight of the unemptied baggage cart contributes to this feeling. Sleep is not the cure for all problems, but it is a key part of the rejuvenation process. As the cart becomes heavier, it takes a toll on your physical, mental, and emotional health, creating a scenario in which your body begins to break down. Our emotional, mental, and physical baggage can break us down, even kill us. We've all heard of people who smoked and drank their way through life yet lived into their 90s, but it's safe to say we've not heard of anyone who's avoided sleep over a prolonged time and lived that long. Sleep is essential. It is the key to your body's repair and rejuvenation process and is one of two (stress being the other) sentinel risk factors that lead to a wide range of other medical conditions.

By choosing to manage your day to get enough sleep, you can actively participate in the daily unloading of your baggage cart. Enhance the degree of restful sleep by staying physically active, avoiding stimulants late in the day (no more 5:00 p.m. runs to the coffeehouse), managing stress, and improving your diet. In this way, sleep becomes productive, allowing for blood transportation and oxygen delivery to the tissues, rejuvenating the body, and making it ready to take on the next day.

LIFESTYLE FACTOR 4: SMOKING

The fourth lifestyle choice for consideration is smoking. Whether or not you smoke plays a significant role in your risk for spinal discomfort. Remember that blood flow and oxygen transport are necessary to maintain healthy tissue. Smoking directly affects the spine on two specific levels. First, smokers are more prone to spinal pain than nonsmokers are because nicotine reduces the flow of blood to the discs, contributing to degenerative changes of the discs. One study showed that blood flow to a lumbar disc was reduced by 50 percent up to one hour after the last cigarette.

Second, smokers have a greater risk for osteoporotic fracture than nonsmokers do because smoking diminishes calcium absorption and prevents new bone growth. Smoking slows recovery after fracture, surgery, or therapy. Nicotine heightens pain perception, so smokers perceive more discomfort than nonsmokers do.

How do your lungs feel when you swim underwater for too long? Your brain gives your muscles a sudden, direct command to get to the surface and take a big breath. When you do, you feel a sense of relief. Without the breath, you feel panic and a sense of urgency. Figuratively, smoking has the same effect on your spinal structures. The tissues become starved for oxygen. A component of spinal pain caused by smoking is the lack of oxygen delivery that leads the tissues to cry out for relief metabolically. They need a big dose of oxygen to feel better.

The effects of smoking on back pain are cumulative. Those who smoke but quit will have to work to rejuvenate the tissues damaged by smoking. The advantage of quitting is that you can begin the process of feeling better without the ongoing negative effects of smoking. You can eat, sleep, and exercise to a healthier spine and happier you.

LIFESTYLE FACTOR 5: STRESS

The final lifestyle concern related to your ability to manage spinal pain is the way in which you manage stress. Good stress management is paramount to helping control a plethora of medical conditions, especially musculoskeletal pain.

Stress is not a completely negative feeling. Good stress, like that generated from activities such as athletic competition, social interaction, and hard work toward personal goals, is called eustress. Among the positive benefits of eustress is the motivation inspired by this stress. How many times have you put off doing something, finally come to grips with the reality that it has to get done, and then completed the task in record time? Eustress can also be helpful in focusing your concentration or enhancing short-burst muscle strength. It improves the immune system and dulls your perception to pain by increasing levels of serotonin in your brain.

Distress, also called controllable stress, arises from our need to control our lives, work, relationships, and so on. It helps us plan, organize, prepare, and follow through on projects.

Uncontrollable stress is the result of events that are beyond our realm of control, such as world politics, an alcoholic spouse, an adult child's failing marriage, or a noisy new neighbor.

The key factor with stress management is the balance of hormones. When we are continually anxious, upset, nervous, frustrated, or angry, the emotional system produces an abundance of the chemical cortisol. Cortisol acts on the blood vessels, causing the smooth muscles lining the walls of the blood vessels to narrow. Blood flow and oxygen delivery to the tissues become more difficult, much as standing on your garden hose limits the flow of water needed to nourish your garden.

Additionally, an overabundance of long-term stress leads to a distortion of restful sleep, an increase of muscle tissue tension (you may refer to them as knots), emotional irritability, and a variety of other situations that may produce symptoms. The American Medical Association estimates that stress is a major component in 90 percent of all illnesses.

Managing stress is easy to say but admittedly hard to do. Consider Joan's story. Joan was experiencing neck pain but could cite no particular incident or trauma that led to the onset of her pain. Her shoulder was beginning to stiffen as well, and she complained of constant headaches. Neck motion was limited, her upper torso muscles were hard, and the discomfort was unremitting. She did not work, instead staying home most of the time with her husband. Treatment led to some relief, but the discomfort gradually returned. Eventually, Joan revealed that she was staying home most of the time to take care of her husband, who had recently become ill. He was no longer working, and Joan was providing care around the clock. She also was dealing with difficult family news from her siblings, and the events had become overwhelming. Joan's sleep had diminished to bouts of a few hours, and she had stopped going to the gym for her weekly exercise class. The physical strain of moving and turning her husband coupled with the emotional strain of the predicament that they were in and the mental strain of the news from her siblings had congealed and located in the muscles of her neck. In physical therapy we acknowledged these issues and how they contributed to her overall level of discomfort. Joan resumed a gym program that incorporated stretches and massages and began to talk about the strain that she was under. She began to report dramatic changes. As Joan started to feel better, her outlook on the situation grew more optimistic. She was able to see that her husband was getting better, his time off work was not permanent, and her own change in roles was going to be temporary as well. Within a few weeks, she was almost back to her old self—sleeping better, moving better, and noting much less discomfort. The neck discomfort that she was experiencing was a symptom of several other factors, not itself a root cause. Stress was the amplifier to her muscles' voice of pain.

Cardiovascular exercise is one of the best ways to manage stress independently. As we described earlier, getting your heart rate into the training zone for 20 to 30 minutes a day can do wonders for hormonal balance. Managing cortisol and increasing levels of dopamine and serotonin through exercise, sleep, diet, and professional help when needed can have a beneficial effect on your level of discomfort regardless of the specific source of the problem.

YOU HAVE CONTROL

The five lifestyle factors described in this chapter are interrelated, either helping or hindering each other. Each can have a positive or negative influence on your level of pain, depending on how you choose to address it. The good thing about these five lifestyle factors is that we have the capacity to manage each of them in a positive way. This is not to say that doing so is always easy, but it can be done. You can exert more influence over your own symptoms than you might have thought. The choice is yours.

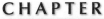

CHAPTER

Learning Correct
Body Mechanics

Sometimes old adages die hard. The advice to bend your knees and lift with your legs to avoid hurting your back is one such adage. Patients, from octogenarians to kids, say this all the time. This statement is correct some of the time, but certainly not all of the time.

In this chapter we argue that you often place more strain on your lower back by bending your knees than by using a different technique. The contrasting photos will show you how different techniques affect the spinal structures when you lift, bend, twist, and reach. The term *body mechanics* refers to the techniques of proper lifting, bending, sweeping, carrying, reaching, and so on. By using appropriate body mechanics, you can reduce the stress and strain on the spinal structures and surrounding muscles, thereby easing discomfort and allowing healing to take place. This discussion of proper body mechanics will teach you how to position and move your body while performing typical work and household tasks so that you experience less discomfort and reduce ongoing irritation and the risk of future injury.

THREE SCENARIOS

To help illustrate the concepts discussed in this chapter, we are going to consider the cases of Paul, Andrea, and Scott. These three cases take into account all the concepts of body mechanics being discussed in this chapter. You will be able to apply these same concepts to the household or work tasks that cause you pain.

Paul was experiencing shoulder pain and chronic neck discomfort on the right side, occasionally radiating to the hand. He expressed concern that his hand was weakening, thereby making it difficult for him to apply the forceful grip to the tools that he used in his work as an electrician. During the evaluation, he revealed that neck extension (looking up) worsened the discomfort. He was in his mid-50s but was in good general health. He was concerned that the arm pain and progressing hand weakness were going to limit his capacity to work. This circumstance was causing him a great deal of stress. To some degree, the problem had been present for several years, but it had recently worsened and occurred at the worst times. He had been working on a large office building in the weeks preceding the flare-up and was anxious about losing his place on that job. "The younger electricians are going to get my work," he worried. "I've got to get back soon." He noted that since seeing his personal doctor about a week before coming to our office, the discomfort had indeed begun to settle. He also noted that he had been taken off work temporarily because of the condition.

Andrea had been having lower back pain that was gradually worsening. Her therapist suspected that her pain originated in the lumbar disc and attributed it to her work at a warehouse, inspecting DVD products as they came off the assembly line. Andrea took the DVDs off the conveyor belt, packaged them, and prepared them for shipping. She was in her mid- to late 20s and not in great physical shape, though not of poor health either. Like many of us, she seemed to have forgotten about the gym. Even with her pain, she was able to do her job without limitation but noted discomfort and difficulty sleeping each night after her shift. Her main complaint was increasing lower back stiffness that made simple tasks such as putting on her shoes uncomfortable. Overall her level of discomfort was worsening. A prior trial of physical therapy had been unsuccessful.

Given the progressive nature of her symptoms, a job site visit was requested. As suspected, the mechanics of her work—not so much what she was doing, but how she was doing it—was provoking her main symptoms. Given a chance to heal, it is likely that her level of discomfort would resolve. Although therapy or medical intervention may have helped her feel better, adjusting how she performed her job was the only thing that would provide lasting, long-term positive results.

Scott was a healthy young man who recently had lumbar fusion surgery. He was self-employed and had been off work for several months, both pre- and postoperatively. He was eager to resume work, given the financial strain that the several months off had caused. His job was to shoe racehorses. As Scott progressed through traditional postsurgical rehab, the focus shifted to back-to-work training. Scott showed the 100-pound (45 kg) anvil that he had to move from the back of his truck to the shoeing site daily. He also demonstrated the horseshoeing position that he used for six hours or more a day. Basically, he had to stand facing away from the horse, bend forward with his elbow on his knee, and hold the horse's leg as he nailed the shoe in place. He used the anvil to shape and adjust the shoe for a proper fit. From a low surface, Scott used a large, heavy mallet to strike the shoe on the anvil while bending forward. The work was often at or below his waist. Scott's problems centered on carrying the heavy anvil to and from the truck each day and bending over to shoe the horse and shape the horseshoe.

Certainly, many other scenarios regarding day-to-day tasks could be used as examples in this discussion of proper body mechanics. Patients frequently mention that loading the dishwasher, lifting cases of water or large bags of dog food, getting items out of the trunk of a car, putting small children into the car seat, changing the linens on the bed, taking out the trash, or cleaning the floors elicits spinal discomfort. The following discussion will help you understand how to do those activities in the proper way to reduce discomfort and keep it from recurring.

FOUR PRIMARY FORCES

Before explaining the concepts of body mechanics and solving the three cases, we need to review the four primary forces that affect muscles and joints during everyday tasks and activities. These forces can lead to tissue strain and pain.

We'll start with compression, a friendly force. The body is well adapted to managing compressive loading forces placed on it. The joints have a thick fibrous covering, the muscles have enough strength capacity to hold us upright against the force of gravity, and the spine is composed of especially large and wide platforms (the vertebral bodies) to bear the weight.

Take your hands and press them firmly together, palm to palm, each point on the left hand contacting a similar point on the right hand (figure 6.1). After maintaining constant pressure for several seconds, do you notice a warmth? A noticeable point of focal pressure? A noticeable area of indentation over part of your hand? A sound? You should have noticed little change in warmth, felt little focal pressure, seen no noticeable indentation on either hand, and heard no sound. In fact, other than using the chest muscles to force the hands together, you should not have sensed much of anything at all.

When you compress your hands together in a parallel position, contact point to contact point, you load your hands in what we call a congruent (equal) manner.

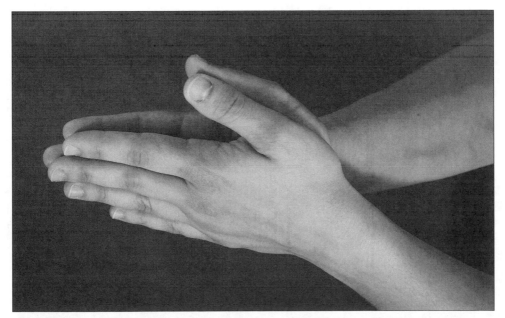

Figure 6.1 Compression force demonstrated by pressing the hands firmly together.

Each point on one hand receives the same amount of pressure as all the points on that hand. The pressure is evenly applied across all parts of both hands. In regard to your spine, this is called axial loading. In general terms, you'd probably call it compression. In either case, congruent axial loading is well tolerated by the body. The joints of your legs and spine are well equipped to maintain their health and function over a long period in such situations.

Consider how you would feel if you placed a large insert into your shoe. Assume that this insert made your left leg about 2 inches (5 cm) longer than the right. You would stand crookedly, your spine would be curved into unusual positions, and the joints of your neck, back, hips, knees, and ankles would bear the weight in unusual and unequal positions. Adding the shoe insert would create an uneven force distribution instead of a symmetrical force alignment. The loading would be absorbed by the joints of the spine and legs in a noncongruent, asymmetrical, and unfamiliar manner.

In truth, compression is not your body's enemy. When compression is applied congruently in aligned positions, the body tolerates it easily. But other destructive forces are at work.

A shear force is a sliding force. To understand shear forces, take your hands and rub them together, moving one hand over the other forward and backward as if you were sanding a piece of wood (figure 6.2). Do you notice a warmth? A feeling of rubbing or wearing through? Are you more aware of your hands than when you simply pressed them together? Do you hear a sound? Is it more apparent that something has happened to your hands now than when you just pressed them together? You likely answered yes to all these questions.

Shear forces are caused when one surface slides over another. Shear forces may occur across all joints of the body. They tend to wear down joints and overtax muscles.

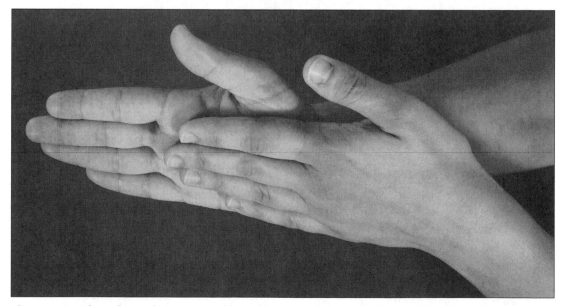

Figure 6.2 Shear force demonstrated by rubbing the hands together in a back and forth motion.

The muscles are responsible for checking these forces, controlling the slide (shear) across the joint surfaces, and promoting a smooth and controlled movement. Your posture correlates to the location of the weight-bearing forces, whether or not it is equal over all aspects of the joint. When the muscles fail to dampen or absorb the shear forces or the position of the joints is not congruent, the joint surface undergoes unwanted and destructive wear and tear similar to what you experienced when you rubbed your hands together.

In the spine, shear force may most easily be understood when you consider what happens when you bend to tie your shoe, pick up a box of tools, lean forward to brush your teeth, or reach above your head to change a light bulb. In these situations, forces are created as if one vertebral segment were sliding over the other. Over time, these shear forces create unwanted joint wear and tear. Arthritic changes, bone spurs, and muscle overuse syndromes are signs of tissue breakdown that eventually leads to pain. Common diagnoses associated with excessive shearing forces include spondylosis, spondylolysthesis, facette arthritis, mechanical spine pain, and muscle overuse syndromes.

Torsion forces are twisting forces. To understand torsion forces, place your hands together and twist them on each other, palm to palm (figure 6.3). Picture what a magician does just before making a coin disappear or what Chubby Checker did with his feet when he sang. Is warmth generated? Do you feel rubbing or wearing?

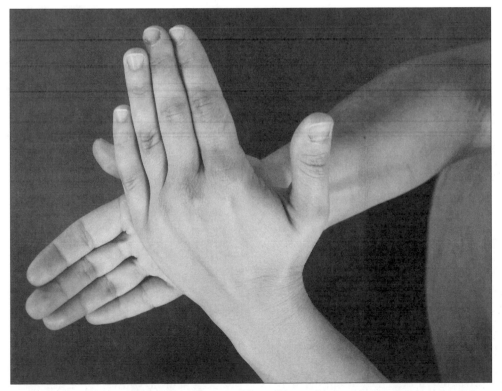

Figure 6.3 Torsion forces demonstrated by rubbing the hands together in a twisting motion.

Do you hear a sound or feel your hands more noticeably than you did when you simply pressed them together? Torsion forces are similar to shear forces except that they occur in the direction of rotation. Health care professionals refer to this as movement in the horizontal, or transverse, plane. You likely call it twisting. When you reach with one hand to open a door, reach behind you to grab the seat belt, or turn your head to back out of the driveway, torsion forces are at play. As with shear forces, muscles are meant to control and check the motion to promote smooth and uniform movement. When motion is excessive or control is poor, torsion forces create unwanted joint trauma, which leads to tissue breakdown and ultimately pain.

The body is designed so that motion gained or lost in one plane will be compensated for by gains or losses in another plane. This idea is easily seen when you watch people walk. (Clinically, we call this gait analysis.) For example, as the arches drop and the legs rotate inward, the pelvis rotates forward and the hips go more into relative flexion. Concurrently, the lumbar spine curve (lordosis) increases. Over time, muscles in the calf and front of the hip shorten while muscles of the abdomen and hip weaken. As these muscles shorten, mobility across the ankles and hips become limited, thereby hindering the overall goal of walking.

As movement is limited, the body compensates, specifically by adding rotation of the lower back. This motion can be observed when watching people walk from behind. Typically, people have a more obvious arm swing, their pelvic girdle moves in a more noticeable front to back motion, and you can often visualize a twisting of the lower lumbar segments back and forth, similar to the hand-to-hand example described earlier. This added lumbar rotation creates localized tissue trauma, leading to a wide variety of clinical symptoms. Because the body is linked as one large chain, the excessive rotation that initially occurs in the feet and is subsequently compensated for at the lumbar region also routinely leads to knee, hip, and even cervical discomfort.

Watch a few people walk, and you will begin to see differences. Most likely these differences are not by choice but are a function of the biomechanics associated with the status of their muscles and joints. Common diagnoses compatible with torsion trauma include disc degeneration, segmental instability, and muscle overuse syndromes.

Just as a woman in pointed high heels would leave an obvious imprint on a freshly seeded lawn compared with another who was wearing wide flat sandals, your joints are similarly affected when one bony surface interfaces with another in a noncongruent, asymmetrical way. Asymmetrical loading also may be demonstrated with the hands. Place the lateral edges of your hands, the sides next to your pinky fingers, firmly together at a 45-degree angle as if cupping your hands to splash water on your face (figure 6.4). What do you feel? Do you notice a focal area of indentation on one hand? Is it more apparent that something has happened to your hands now than when you just pressed them together? Are some parts of your hand under different pressure than other parts? You likely answered yes to all questions. Although you will feel no difference in warmth and hear no sound, the forces associated with asymmetrical loading are just as deleterious as shear and torsion forces.

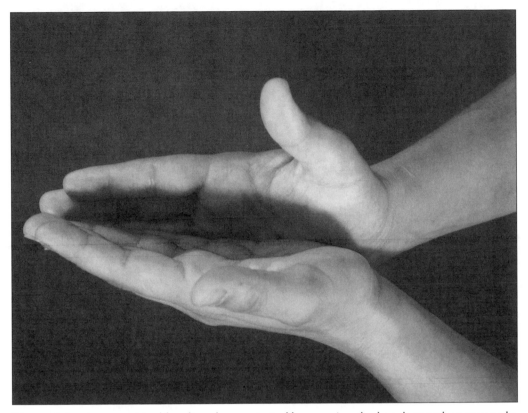

Figure 6.4   Asymmetrical loading demonstrated by pressing the hands together unevenly.

Because the same pressure of force is being applied to less surface area, you will likely agree that there is more pressure on each aspect of your hand, producing a greater feeling of compression.

Over time the surrounding tissues become overloaded, irritated, and either shortened or lengthened, depending on which side of the asymmetry they are on. The joint surfaces and surrounding tissues begin to break down. What we refer to as localized tissue irritation you likely call pain.

Asymmetrical loading in the lower spine is common when the spinal curve is larger than appropriate (for example, an exaggerated lordosis) or when a side bend issue is present because of a leg length inequality. In the upper spine, asymmetrical loading may be caused when an awkward bending of the neck occurs over a long period (for example, when constantly on the phone without a head set or when constantly looking down to type or sew). Asymmetrical loading in the spine is a common culprit with diagnoses of facette syndromes, mechanical spine pain, stenosis, disc bulges, and arthritis.

One other force applied across the spine is distraction. This pulling-apart force often is applied intentionally in a therapeutic manner in an effort to unload or uncompress a problem area. Your doctor or therapist may refer to traction, which implies treatment to help ease the discomfort and stretch the involved area.

BODY MECHANIC TECHNIQUES

Medication and therapy will not permanently solve your back and neck pain if you continue to expose your body to the factors that led to the problem in the first place. Using the body mechanic techniques described in this chapter is the best way to reduce the harmful shear, torsion, and asymmetrical loading strains that break down tissue and lead to pain. In a clinical setting, the clinician can use demonstrations and words to help a patient understand proper body mechanics. In this chapter, we will rely on photos to demonstrate how to reduce unwanted spinal forces and ease spinal pain during day-to-day activities and work-related tasks.

The three primary concepts are the following:

1. Use whole-body movements that incorporate weight shifts.
2. Use the larger muscles and joints of the hips and shoulders rather than the smaller muscles and joints of the back and neck.
3. Keep the work or item close to you.

Applying these three concepts is as simple as doing one thing: using a stagger stance.

Technique 1: Stagger Stance

When in a stagger stance (figure 6.5), one foot will be slightly ahead of the other. You may stand with your feet a normal width apart, but you place one foot about one-half of a foot length ahead of the other.

The stagger stance will allow you to shift your weight forward and backward for activities such as vacuuming, sweeping, raking, or reaching overhead to put away dishes, trim tree branches, or paint. Maintaining a slight stagger stance will even make

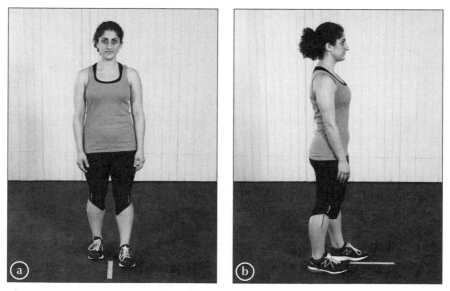

Figure 6.5   Stagger stance: *(a)* front view; *(b)* side view.

simple activities such as standing in line easier. You will be more comfortable when you wash the dishes, stand to prepare food, lift things from the floor, brush your teeth, shave, or put on makeup.

Using a stagger stance is one of the two primary techniques that we emphasize. The stagger stance takes a considerable amount of strain off the neck and lower lumbar spine by promoting a more neutral (balanced) pelvic girdle position. The larger shoulder and hip muscles support the body, rather than just the smaller muscles and joints of the spine. The stagger stance facilitates shifting your weight so that you can keep items close to you and reduce the load on the spine.

A stagger stance allows you to reach overhead with less shoulder and neck strain. When the feet are side by side, all forward-reaching movements require an equal force generated by the back muscles to maintain a balanced upright position (figure 6.6a). The farther forward that you reach, the greater the demand is on the spine. A weight of 10 pounds (4.5 kg) at your side may require a trunk muscular force of 100 pounds (45 kg) to counteract that weight as you reach forward. The stagger stance (figure 6.6b) allows you to shift your weight forward as you reach forward, effectively keeping the item closer to you and minimizing the counterbalance needed. The neck and shoulder muscles work far easier when the body is in the stagger stance position than when the feet are side by side.

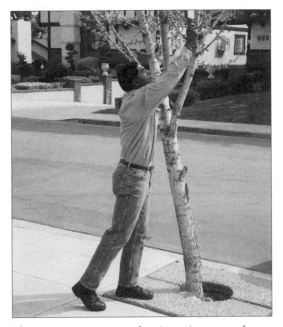

The stagger stance makes it easier to perform overhead activities.

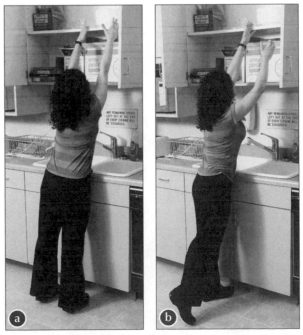

Figure 6.6 Reaching overhead with (a) feet side by side and (b) with feet staggered.

The stagger stance position promotes lifting from the floor with your knees out of the way (figure 6.7a). When you are lifting items from the floor, the stagger stance positions your knees at a diagonal and out of the way, allowing you to keep the item closer to you. Whether the knees are bent or not doesn't matter; the key is to keep them out of the way so the item is closer to you. When the feet are side by side (figure 6.7b), you have to reach beyond your knees to grasp the item. This stance places the torso in a more horizontal position, which strains the spine. When the feet are staggered, the hands end up well inside the knees and the angle of the torso is more vertical, allowing the head to stay up.

To get an idea of the difference that keeping the item close to you makes, hold a bag of groceries in each hand with your forearms jutting forward and your elbows bent at the side. Now reach forward with both bags with your elbows straight in front of you. Which arm position is better for carrying the groceries? Compare the difference. Intuitively, we know that having the groceries closer to the body is easier, and that's how we naturally carry things. You don't walk in the garden with the shovel pointing straight in front of you. Rather, you grasp it in the middle with the shaft at your side. The same concept applies to lifting things from the floor. The more vertical your spine is, the easier it will be.

When you mop, rake, shovel, vacuum, or sweep, the stagger stance allows you to shift your weight from side to side or front to back, keeping the mop, rake, shovel, vacuum, or broom in concert with your front hand. By moving the front foot in the direction that you want to work, you keep the spine generally torsion free while your hips rotate. When the front hand moves beyond the front foot, the strain on the spine increases substantially. Shifting your weight as you work gives you the advantage of using your whole body to apply the sweeping, shoveling, or mopping force.

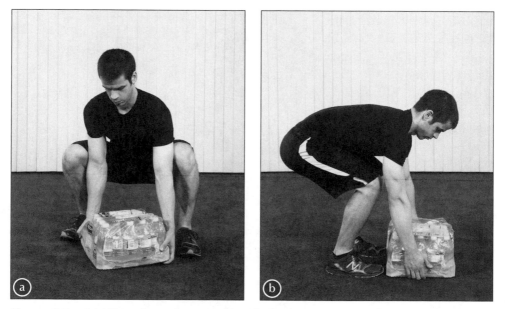

Figure 6.7   (a) Lifting from the ground with the feet in staggered stance. (b) Lifting from the ground with the feet side by side.

Visualize a worker shoveling debris. Back bent, feet side by side, he or she bends to scoop up a load of dirt, fully loading the spine. Upon returning to an upright position, again placing full demand on the spine, he or she twists to the side to dump the dirt into a wheelbarrow (figure 6.8a). This extra torsion force gradually but greatly wears down the discs, eventually causing pain. By using a stagger stance, the worker could shift his or her weight onto the forward foot when scooping up the dirt (figure 6.8b), shift onto the back foot when returning to upright, and then take a drop step similar to a basketball player's pivot to move the whole body to the right to deposit the debris (figure 6.8c). Can you appreciate the difference in shear and torsion forces on the spine in these examples? The same is true for any similar task.

The stagger stance allows you to accomplish all three of our primary concepts whether you are lifting, reaching forward, carrying, sweeping, mopping, or raking.

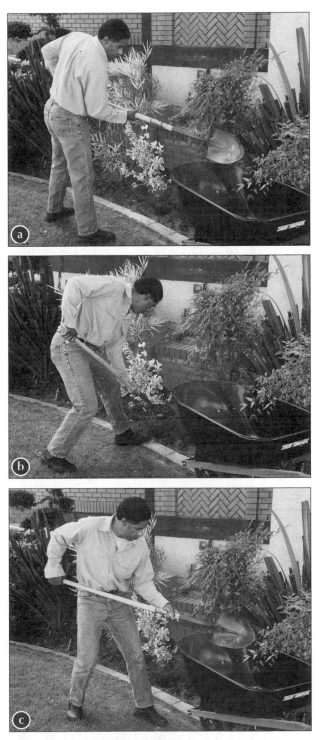

Figure 6.8 Shoveling debris into a wheelbarrow: (a) feet side by side, which places too much stress on the spine; (b) feet in stagger stance, which allows the worker to shift his weight onto the forward foot when digging then (c) shift onto the back foot and pivot to deposit the debris into the wheelbarrow.

Myth

I MUST BEND MY KNEES WHEN I LIFT

When lifting, the most important factor to consider is how to keep the item close to you. If bending your knees accomplishes this, then bend your knees when you lift. But if bending your knees puts the item farther away than necessary, don't bend your knees. In this case, bending your knees will make the lift harder and put more strain on your back.

The important point is to get your knees out of the way when you lift. To do this, you need to use a stagger stance and the golfer's lift.

Also important is keeping the item close. Imagine how difficult it would be to carry groceries by holding the bags at shoulder height and arm's length. When bending the knees to lift, we often position ourselves too far from the item to be moved, increasing the stress on the spine. Bending the knees isn't necessarily what makes the lift safe or not. The important point is where you position yourself and where the item is when you begin the task. Using the stagger stance and golfer's lift allows you to keep the items close and use weight shifts to move the object safely.

Technique 2: Golfer's Lift

The golfer's lift (figure 6.9) is a straight leg (or generally so) version of the stagger stance in which you move to lift, grab, place, or position an item with one or both hands while letting one foot gently glide back and up off the ground, similar to the way in which a golfer retrieves the ball from the cup. You do not need to lift the back leg far off the ground. The action is far easier than that. Simply allow the back foot to slide back while you reach forward, up, or laterally. The back foot need only lightly touch the ground. This movement unlocks your hip joint, allowing motion there while shifting the demand off your spine. If necessary, brush your hand against

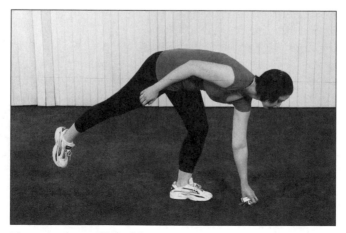

Figure 6.9 Golfer's lift.

a wall, lean the thigh of your standing leg against a cabinet, or place your hand on a nearby object to help you balance.

Picture yourself leaning over a table to serve a hot dish, reaching to lift a small bathroom wastebasket, bending over to make the bed, or picking up a bucket full of tools. Imagine leaning over the trunk to lift out the spare tire, bending to wash your face or brush your teeth, lifting a bucket of soapy water by the handle to wash the car, or grabbing your briefcase or purse off the ground. Simply allow your back leg to slide back and slightly up off the floor. This movement shifts the demand directly to your hips and recruits the larger gluteal and hamstring muscles to control the movement, rather than the smaller muscles of the spine. Use the golfer's lift to grab small items such as keys or shoes off the floor and for reaching larger, heavier items as well.

The weight of the item doesn't matter. Lifting a 50-pound (23 kg) paint can with one arm in a bent-over golfer's lift is far easier than squatting, grabbing the can, and standing up again in a bend-your-knees lift. The goal is to keep the item close to you. The golfer's lift places you directly over the item that you wish to retrieve, keeping it as close as possible and subsequently requiring the least effort. When two hands are needed to lift the object, use the stagger stance lift (page 102). When one hand will do, consider working the golfer's lift into your routine.

Use this technique to get items out of a low cupboard or the dishwasher. Rather than stoop from a distance or squat or kneel all the way down, simply face the countertop, use one hand for balance, and use the other hand to get the item. Approach from the side so that you can see into the cupboard or dishwasher better. Let the back leg, the leg opposite the hand that you use to pick up the object, drift slightly back and up

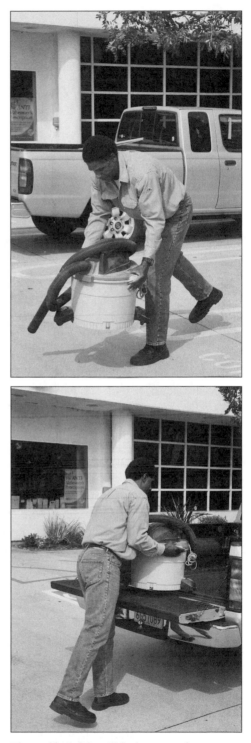

The golfer's lift will help you when you have to pick up a heavy bucket off the ground or pull something out of the back of a truck.

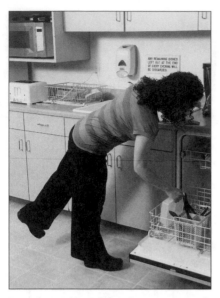

Use the golfer's lift when you need to retrieve items from the dishwasher or a low cabinet.

off the floor. You can twist, reach, and bend to get things from a low or back shelf easily this way. The technique may feel different at first, but it should not be painful. With a little practice and time, you'll agree that the golfer's lift solves more problems than it creates.

You may be thinking, "They've described two techniques that redirect the forces to the hips. Won't my hips wear out?" Or maybe you already have bad hips. Don't worry. By design, the hip joints are deep seated, well muscled, and built for stability. If your hips are not hurting now, these techniques will not wear them out. If your hips already hurt, efficient movements that create less strain aren't going to add to the pain. In fact, you may find that your aching knees also benefit as you maximize your body as a whole while minimizing forces directed at one joint alone.

Technique 3: Push, Don't Pull

When at all possible, push, don't pull (figure 6.10). Pushing accomplishes each of the three main concepts. To move a sofa, slide a piece of furniture, get behind the bed, roll a large bin, mow the lawn, or do any specific work task, pushing is always better. Note that you want to position yourself on the diagonal corner of the object as opposed to the middle if possible.

Picture a table in the middle of a room. To slide the table forward a few feet (a meter), you have several choices. You can stand beside the table and slide it in the direction that you want to go, you can get at one end and pull it toward you, or you can stand at the other end and push it forward. The first choice is the least desirable, because you have to twist your spine in the direction that you want to move the table, creating way too much torsion force. The second choice is a little better, but it requires you to pull. The third choice is best. All you have to do is shift your weight in the direction that you want to go and the table will move.

Even better is to stand at the corner of the table. This position allows you to use a weight shift from a stagger stance, one thigh pressing against the edge of the table and the front foot simply waiting for the weight to shift onto it. You can move refrigerators, couches, washing machines, and tables with minimal effort of the hands and back simply by standing on the diagonal and using your thighs to weight shift the object a small distance at a time. After the object is out in the open, get in the middle and give it a push to move it where you want.

Pushing requires nothing more than leaning into the object and driving with your strong leg muscles. When you pull, the trouble begins because your legs and arms end up parallel in one plane and your torso is working hard to keep them together

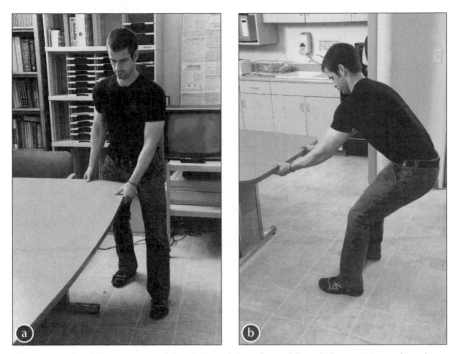

Figure 6.10   To move a table, *(a)* pushing the table while positioned at the diagonal corner of the table is a better option than *(b)* pulling the table.

in another plane. Usually, the legs and arms are more parallel to the floor and the torso tends to be more vertical. This technique requires a lot of effort from the trunk muscles to hold the two together. Because many of us have diminished strength, the forces are directed to the small ligaments, discs, and tissues of the spine rather than the large muscle groups of the thighs and shoulders.

If you have to pull, position yourself so that the arms, legs, and torso are generally aligned in the same direction. As you lean back, you should be in a stagger stance so that you are essentially falling in the direction that you want to move. Hold onto the item as you fall and back it will go. In this way, all the forces needed to move the item are aligned in a straight line passing through you, requiring much less muscular effort to control. If you do pull, the goal is to have your arms, legs, and torso pointing in the same direction.

Because shifting your weight and using the hips and upper back is important for all these body mechanics techniques, you can understand why we spent so much time in the exercise section on those areas.

APPLYING GOOD BODY MECHANICS

Now that we've discussed shear, torsion, and asymmetrical loading forces and the primary concepts and techniques for proper positioning and movement, let's return to our three cases to see whether we can apply these principles to Paul, Andrea, and Scott.

Reaching Overhead

Paul is the middle-aged electrician who reported progressive right arm pain and weakness, especially when he looked up. A review of his work techniques made several things clear. When he worked overhead, Paul routinely stood flat footed with his feet side by side, stressing and straining to tighten, hold, turn, or fasten various things. He seldom used a foot ladder, not even a small step stool, even though one was readily available. The recent flare-up coincided with a change in the progression of the job. In the last several weeks, he had moved to doing more overhead tasks. By incorporating a stagger stance when he worked overhead, he was able to gain some extension through his upper back and hips, thereby reducing it from his neck. Paul soon could feel and see the difference between a flat-footed stance and a stagger stance. Placing one foot on a small portable step stool allowed him to reduce looking up still further. Although he could not do all his work in these better positions, by the end of the workday he had a much smaller amount of the cumulative irritation compared with what he had felt in the previous weeks. Reducing neck extension led to a more open cervical foramen and less irritation of the nerve root within the bony walls of the tunnel. Paul added mobility activities for the upper thoracic spine and general fitness and conditioning of the postural muscles and was able to return to work and finish the job. If he hadn't changed his positions and movement patterns, it's likely that Paul would have continued to experience pain and limitations in his ability to work.

Think of a task that you do that requires continual or repetitive overhead activity, such as painting, trimming trees, or rearranging your kitchen shelves. Use a slight stagger stance and allow your weight to shift forward and back or side to side with the needs of the job. You'll find your tasks a whole lot easier to do and less stressful to the neck and lower back.

Bending and Twisting

Andrea worked at a DVD plant inspecting, packaging, and preparing DVDs for shipment. Standing with her feet side by side at the conveyor belt, Andrea repetitively bent to grab items and then twisted to sort them into bins. At another station, she took packaged boxes and moved them left or right into different piles. Lifting from the floor on her left, she often had to stack the boxes off to the left. At a different station, she sat for hours boxing products, reaching forward to clear the sort bin in front of her many times during a shift. The golfer's lift was the best technique for Andrea. By allowing her trailing leg to drift slightly back and up off the floor, Andrea was able to lean over the conveyor belt without straining the lumbar discs and muscles. Additionally, this technique allowed her to twist and rotate to grab items as they passed by or drop them into different bins, moving at the hip rather than the fixed torso. When she moved to the sorting and shipping area, Andrea used a diagonal stance with the knees out of the way when she lifted the boxes and then transitioned to the golfer's lift. This method let her move her weight into the right direction without planting her feet and twisting her spine. When she had to pick boxes off storage shelves and place them on a rolling cart, she again used the golfer's lift. She was easily able to lift each box with two hands and maintain her balance because the back foot was just in contact with the floor behind her. After she had the box, the lift promoted the use of the hamstrings, not the smaller paraspinous muscles, to assist in returning to the upright position. Minimizing torsion, especially in a forward bent position, greatly reduced the irritation of the lumbar tissues and disc. Within a week or so the problem began to subside noticeably, and Andrea was well on her way to meeting her rehab goals.

Imagine a task that you do at home or at the office that requires bending forward and moving side to side. In a sense, Andrea's job was similar to what you do when you bend over to unload the dishwasher, take groceries out of the cart to place them on the checkout belt, or move luggage out of the trunk. Leaning forward with a golfer's lift followed by movement side to side, each leg coming ever so slightly off the ground, allows for movement in all directions without lumbar stress and strain.

Lifting and Bending

Scott had the unique job of shoeing horses. After he returned to work, he had the task of carrying a 100-pound (45 kg) anvil from his truck to the job site. Then he had to bend over to shoe the horse for five minutes or longer at a time, four times for each horse, eight or so horses a day. First, Scott had to learn to slide the anvil off the back of his truck. Scott's choice was to stand at the corner of the truck bed and lean back to slide the anvil to the edge. He found it easy to stand with his feet staggered and simply shift his weight from the front foot to the back to move the anvil. Next he had to lift the anvil out of the truck bed and lower it onto the low sawhorses he used for a table. Lowering the weight between his knees rather than in front of his knees was the trick. By keeping his feet wide and slightly staggered, he could keep the knees out of the way and keep his back vertical while he moved the anvil toward the table. Next, he had to figure out how to shoe the horses without straining his surgically repaired back. This took some adjustment. To maintain the positioning principles, Scott leaned onto his knee with his elbow, acting as his own brace, thus minimizing the muscular demand on the paraspinal muscles of the back. Although he remained bent over, he was passively supporting his weight rather than relying on the muscles to do so for him. This technique is perfect for changing the sheets on a bed, bending to pick up the morning paper, or fixing something low to the ground. We incorporated the repetitive back bending described in chapter 4 in addition to a good fitness program that counteracted the repeated bending that he did. Scott was able to resume work, tolerate some recreation, and generally resume life without major limitation. Despite any well-intentioned intervention, had Scott returned to work using the same positions and movements that preceded his surgery, he would not have experienced the success provided by the training in body mechanics.

Imagine activities that you do at home or work that require constant bending. Perhaps your job requires a lot of sitting. Add some golf or biking, both forward-flexed activities, on the weekend, spend a little time at the computer or TV during the week, and the next thing you know you've got neck or back pain. The key is to examine as a whole the positions and movements of all your tasks and determine which ones are making you hurt. Often you'll find that if you can implement techniques to minimize shear, torsion, and asymmetrical loading forces, you can reduce discomfort without any other intervention at all.

This chapter has covered some basic concepts and techniques to make daily tasks easier and less straining. Initially, these techniques may feel a bit odd, but with a little practice you'll find that they fit as well as your favorite pair of shoes. They help you feel more comfortable, and you can take them anywhere.

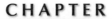

Adapting Office Ergonomics

By definition, ergonomics refers to the study of work, that is, how the body performs work and the effect that work has on the body. In the teaching of office ergonomics, much like the teaching of body mechanics in chapter 6, we are really trying to show you how to work smarter, not harder. Given today's high-tech, computer-dominant world, in which sitting for prolonged periods at work is often followed by sitting for prolonged periods at home, the setup of your computer workstation can play a large factor in your ability to stay symptom free.

You may have had multiple treatments for your discomfort. Has your therapist or doctor given you the impression that you've tried everything from A to Z, up and down, and still you return complaining of neck, upper back, and shoulder pain? What else can you do?

Whoever coined the phrase "experience is the best teacher" was certainly correct. With over a hundred treatment years combined, we know exactly where the answer lies. Those lingering aches and pains are no longer such a mystery.

For many with spinal pain, the solution lies not with an isolated treatment by a doctor, therapist, or acupuncturist. Rather, the solution to ease those ongoing and lingering complaints of neck and lower back discomfort often rests in your hands and those of your company's employee health and safety director, maintenance crew, or office manager. Even your own family members at home play a part. Anyone responsible for adjusting heights, ordering supplies, and changing alignments of the computer work area is key. After finishing this chapter you will be able to assess and adjust your computer work area to achieve the overall goal of easing your neck and back discomfort.

In this chapter we'll discuss how the positioning of your workstation, your posture at the workstation, and the techniques that you use while working greatly affect your ability to stay symptom free. You will be able to analyze your own work area and decide what positional, equipment, and technique changes are necessary to improve your comfort.

Those with nagging neck, upper back, shoulder, arm, and lower back pain should understand that these complaints often result from factors that are not quickly cured with an injection, simple stretch, or isolated exercise. To achieve a lasting remedy, we need to disrupt the causative factors and eliminate the irritating events that lead up to the symptoms. Only then will you notice full and lasting success.

FATIGUE TO DISABILITY CONTINUUM

The concept of the fatigue to disability continuum (figure 7.1) is useful to our discussion because it helps demonstrate how conditions and their resulting symptoms develop over time. What you initially notice as heaviness or fatigue will, if left unchecked, become obvious discomfort. If left unchecked, the discomfort will lead to pain. If left unchecked, the pain will worsen, resulting in an injury that, if left unattended, will ultimately lead to disability. As you can see, given the same set of circumstances, over time the severity of the condition will worsen.

In various chapters, we've discussed the physiological and biomechanical concepts relating to fitness and strength, cellular health and resiliency, body posture, and positioning, among others. In this chapter on office ergonomics, those concepts come together to form the framework of our ergonomic message: Over time, static posturing in a poor position combined with repetitive movements leads to a predictable series of events. Therefore, in regard to working at your desk or on your computer, understand that the discomfort and pain that you feel are not the result of one-time events. Rather, they occur over time because of repeated exposure. A gradual breakdown of tissue tolerance leads to a predictable series of events. The fatigue to disability continuum provides a roadmap of what to expect.

Many years of traveling to work sites to evaluate employees who complained of discomfort revealed three trends. Employees reporting discomfort had similar faults in their computer area setups. In situations in which people were not complaining of symptoms, the same poor findings frequently were noted. The fatigue to disability continuum suggested that although some employees may not have been experiencing symptoms yet, the wheels had been set in motion. It was only a matter of time until they began to hurt. Also apparent was that those who were generally more fit tended to be the ones not yet complaining of discomfort, and those of less overall fitness seemed to be already reporting tissue breakdown (pain) even though both had similarly poor workstation setups.

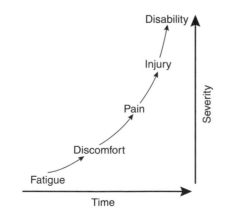

Figure 7.1   Fatigue to disability continuum.

WORK AREA TRENDS THAT CAUSE PAIN

The three common workstation trends that predictably lead to the onset of neck, midback, arm, or leg symptoms are overreaching, using incorrect heights, and maintaining an unbalanced work area (table 7.1). Let's look at each of these individually before learning to analyze and adjust your work area. You'll need to understand these three concepts to be able to identify them in your situation and take corrective action. You can't change what you can't see or don't recognize.

Table 7.1   Three Workstation Trends and Their Effects

	Overreaching	Incorrect heights	Unbalanced work area
Shoulder tendinitis or impingement	Keyboard, mouse, and 10-key too far away; armrests in the way		
Nerve compression (carpal tunnel)		Chair, keyboard, or desktop wrong height or not adjustable	Phone, mouse, and desktop items all on the same side
Muscle spasm, tightness in the neck and shoulders	Keyboard, mouse, and 10-key too far away; armrests in the way		
Lateral epicondylitis (tennis elbow)	Keyboard, mouse, and 10-key too far away; armrests in the way		Phone, mouse, and desktop items all on the same side
Overuse syndromes or repetitive motion injury			Phone, mouse, and desktop items all on the same side
Neck compression, rotation, or stenosis dysfunctions		Monitor or chair at the wrong height	Monitor not centered; copy work not centered

Overreaching

Overreaching refers to the horizontal axis, that is, a plane parallel to the floor. Common diagnoses associated with overreaching at a computer workstation include shoulder tendinitis, impingement, elbow lateral epicondylitis (tennis elbow), and muscle spasm and tightness in the lateral neck and midback.

Overreaching refers to the position of items on the desktop such as a keyboard, 10-key numeric keypad, mouse, binders and documents, fax machines, phones, staplers, and other desk equipment (figure 7.2). Overreaching is a common finding when the mouse and keyboard are not positioned on the same surface, when the armrests on the chair do not lower to fit beneath the desktop or drop-down keyboard tray, or when the arrangement of items on the desk is not appropriate. For example, some people place papers on the front edge of the desk and then reach past them to type and enter data. Often the keyboard will be on a drop-down tray, but the mouse will be up on the desktop a full arm's length away.

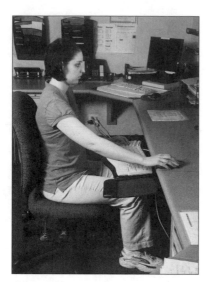

Figure 7.2 Examples of over-reaching on a common desktop.

Most overreaching issues are easily correctable. Simply rearranging the desktop or purchasing inexpensive products seems to solve many of these ergonomic setup concerns rather quickly.

In the body mechanics chapter, we discussed the importance of keeping items close to you. In regard to ergonomics, when you overreach you place repeated and unnecessary muscle strain on the larger muscles of the neck, shoulder, and upper back while simultaneously increasing the demand on the smaller muscles of the hands, forearm, and shoulder. Over time, these larger muscles become overactive, resulting in spasms and restrictions, often called knots. The smaller muscles tire, eventually breaking down and leading to tendinitis. In both cases, you end up with discomfort.

One obvious overreaching case involved an employee who had to scan and fax hundreds of bills each day for processing. While seated at the computer, she had to upload data from a paper bill and then lean across to her right to scan and fax it. She did this all day, processing hundreds of bills each shift. Without a change in the reaching aspect of the job, no treatment option would have any lasting success in mitigating her pain. The predictable outcome for what was initially reported as pain would progress to injury and eventually lead to disability.

Evaluating Overreaching

Assess your workstation:

- Are the keyboard and mouse on the same surface?
- Is the mouse close to the keyboard?
- Do the armrests prevent you from sliding your chair all the way under the desktop or keyboard tray?
- Are commonly used items such as binders, keyboard, 10-key numeric keypad, and phone close to you?
- Do you use a document holder?
- Do you have a hands-free headset and a feature that allows you to answer the phone by striking a computer key?
- Does the chair fit you? Is the seat pan, the part that you sit on, too deep, or is the backrest not adjustable?
- Are the proper items in each of the proper zones?

Using Incorrect Heights

Incorrect height refers to the vertical axis, that is, a plane perpendicular to the ground. Common diagnoses associated with the use of incorrect heights include nerve compression syndromes, most often at the wrist, and neck compression problems including stenosis (narrowing of the neural tunnel) and facette joint dysfunctions. Of the three, this one most often leads to lower back problems as well, aggravating a disc issue if the chair is too low and worsening a stenosis issue if the chair is too high.

Incorrect height may involve the positioning of the chair, including the armrests, seat back, seat pan, the desktop where your work is placed, the monitor, and the surface holding the keyboard and mouse (figure 7.3). In many cases, several users are assigned to each computer station. Many of us have this difficulty at home. Mom and dad share the computer, and kids of varying ages vie for time to do homework and play games. In neither case is the setup perfectly correct for any one user; rather, some aspects are good for the adults and other aspects good for the kids. This common problem occurs when multiple users share a work area.

Incorrect height may also be related to furniture and features of the work area that are not adjustable. In many cases, companies initially purchase furniture that is adjustable to accommodate multiple users as they come and go within the department or division. Other work areas tend to materialize out of necessity and unforeseen events. These setups lack the adjustability necessary to accommodate various users. Often keyboards will be on standard height desktops and monitors will be far too high or low to promote any degree of comfort. Home workstations often lack the sophistication of their office counterparts. Reams of paper serve as makeshift monitor risers, egg crates serve as footrests, and a child's old play table ends up supporting the keyboard or mouse. Do any of these examples pertain to you? Incorrect heights

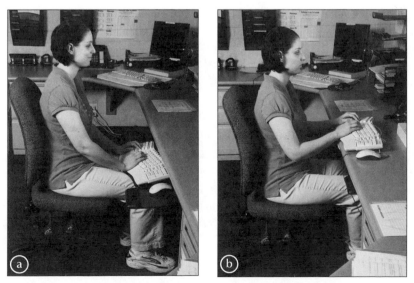

Figure 7.3 Example of incorrect heights at a common workstation: *(a)* Keyboard is too low; *(b)* keyboard is too high.

are more difficult to correct than the other two ergonomic culprits. Of critical importance is the chair, which we'll discuss more fully in a few pages.

Trina's case demonstrates the relevance of workstation height. Trina complained of nervelike symptoms starting in her right wrist. She also had shoulder and arm pain and stiffness in her neck. She was just above 5 feet (152 cm) tall and had a small frame. She had moved to that work area about six months earlier. She had begun to notice the symptoms about four weeks before the evaluation and reported that her symptoms were definitely worsening. Although she didn't know who had used the cubicle space before her, one of her cubicle mates did. As suspected, the man who had previously inhabited the cubicle was tall, nearly 6 feet, 5 inches (196 cm). The work area was pretty much as he had left it. Trina had been working in a location set up for someone nearly 17 inches (43 cm) taller than she was. The chair was far too large for her, and the desktop was set above the usual height. The monitor position was nearly 12 inches (30 cm) too tall for her even with the chair all the way up. By constantly looking up, Trina was compressing the neural tunnel and smashing the nerve root at the neck in addition to placing unwanted pressure on the nerve at the wrist. Unbeknown to her, the nerve was being compressed from both ends. After a massive readjustment of the workspace in which the desktop was lowered and a drop-down keyboard tray and footrest were added, among others changes, Trina began to improve gradually and steadily. Naturally, she was happy as she began to feel better and didn't have to miss work. Her employer was pleased as well. The power of an ergonomic assessment was in full display.

Does this situation resemble what you deal with at work? Did you inherit a work area, or are you using a work area that was put together without regard to who was going to use it? If so, your spinal discomforts may not be as complicated to fix as you may think.

Evaluating Height

Assess your workstation:

- Is the chair adjustable (the seat pan, backrest, and armrests)?
- Is the desktop height adjustable? Can you raise or lower the entire surface?
- Is your workstation one continuous piece all at the same height, or are there pieces with sections to accommodate different tasks (typing, writing, reading)?
- Is the top line of the text as displayed on the monitor at eye level? If you wear bifocals, the top line of the text as displayed on the monitor should be 2 inches (5 cm) lower than eye level.

Unbalanced Work Area

An unbalanced work area refers to the transverse, or rotational, plane. Common diagnoses associated with an unbalanced work area include neural compression syndromes, overuse and repetitive motion syndromes at the shoulder and elbow, and neck compression syndrome.

An unbalanced work area most often refers to the position of the items on your desktop (figure 7.4). About 87 percent of the population is right-handed. Issues arise when the right hand is used for all desktop activities such as using the mouse, answering the phone, using the 10-key pad, grasping binders or file folders, and so on. Many desks have just such a setup. It's no wonder that many of us end up with right-sided shoulder, neck, elbow, or nerve pain. The other common finding is an off-center position of the monitor. As you analyze your desk area, consider the layout of your items. Chances are that you'll be able to move some of them to the left or move the monitor to the center. The solution is often to place items such as the phone, stapler, binders, mouse, pens, papers, and the like to the side opposite where they are now.

The phone is almost always the first item that you should move. Because most of us reach with the right arm and then quickly transfer the receiver over to the left to use the right hand to write a note or number, why not simply begin the process with the left hand and give the right side a bit of a reprieve?

Another common culprit is the position of the monitor. It should be central to your line of view, aligned directly in front of you. If you're having neck discomfort, a slightly offset computer monitor is likely part of the source of your symptoms. Moving it to the center makes a large difference.

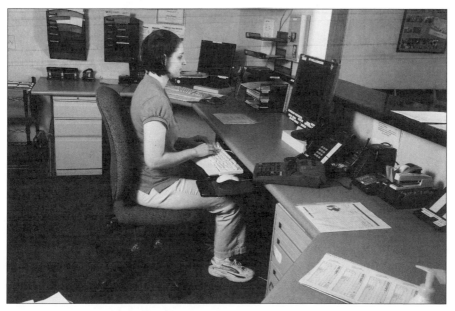

Figure 7.4   An unbalanced work area.

As a manager, Molly held occasional meetings with several employees at a time. They were asked to sit at her desk in front of her. Molly's job primarily involved working on the computer. As a manager, her desk and chair were more stylish than those of the general working crew, appropriate for meeting with people. To be able to see her staff at these weekly 20- to 30-minute meetings, she located her monitor off center to her right. Her main complaints were worsening headaches and neck pain on the right side. She complained of stiffness when she turned her head to the right. The discomfort was local and did not travel into her arm. At first glance, the solution appeared to be simple. In choosing to accommodate face-to-face contact for a weekly 30-minute meeting, she had chosen to make the other 45 hours or more a week that she spent at her desk miserable by placing her monitor significantly off to the right. By relocating her phone lines to the left, switching the monitor to the center of the desk, and moving the guest chairs to either side of her monitor, we quickly and cheaply improved the work area ergonomics to promote a more comfortable work experience. Everyone could see each other during the weekly meetings, and Molly's head was straight forward during the remainder of her workweek.

The point is that these adjustments usually aren't complicated or tricky, and they often have a significant effect on the level of discomfort that you may feel. Within 20 minutes the problem was identified, a solution suggested, and adjustments implemented. One week later Molly reported that she had excellent success. What amount of medication or therapy could resolve her problem as simply or completely as resolving the initial cause of the symptom in the first place? Until the offset computer monitor was moved, the symptoms could not resolve.

Evaluating an Unbalanced Work Area

Assess your workstation:

- Are the majority of desktop items off to the same side?
- Do you have commonly used items closest to you and reference items and fax machines farthest from you?
- Is your monitor centered on your desk, directly in line with your direction of view?
- Do you use a 10-key pad or other specialty tool? Is it located on the same side as your phone and mouse?

ARRANGING YOUR OFFICE

Success always begins with a good plan. Whether you are setting up a home office for the first time or moving into an existing work space, planning where to put things makes a big difference in your overall long-term level of comfort. Consider the following concepts.

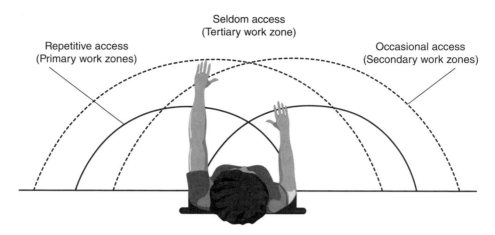

Figure 7.5 Where to put desktop items: the three zones of reference.

First, the layout of the room often determines the layout of the desktop items. For example, some people do not want their backs to the office door or their papers facing a window where others could easily view them. They set up their office work area backward, trying to fit the monitor and keyboard placement to the furniture rather than moving the furniture to get the best overall alignment. If you're moving into an area and have a specific need to sit in one direction or another, expend some short-term effort to coordinate your moving in with the position and layout of the furniture as you want it to be. If you don't do this, long-term discomfort may be on the way.

Second, consider placing items in such a way that you have to get up out of the chair periodically to use them. For example, copiers, faxes, printers, and so on can be located either down the hall or outside your immediate desk area. If they are close to you, be sure that they are at least an arm's length or two away. This arrangement forces you to get up out of the chair, disrupting the deleterious effects of long-term static positioning that so often contribute to symptoms. This intentional standing period is called a microbreak. More than a few of the desk areas that we've seen have a fax or copy machine so close that the user could simply reach across to use it. Refer to the diagram that illustrates where to put desktop items, as recommended by the Occupational Safety & Health Administration (figure 7.5). Notice the three zones of reference. Consider your own workstation setup. Does it follow this recommended model?

Desktop Items

The primary desktop zone is where your day-to-day items go, the ones that you use all day long, such as pens and papers; keyboard and mouse; sewing, drafting, or drawing tools; phone; calculator; paperwork; and so on. These items should all be within easy reach, balanced equally on both sides.

The secondary zone is for those items used daily, but not necessarily all day. For example, reference binders and manuals are items that you may use every day for a short time but not again for some time. These types of items should not occupy primary desk space and should be relegated to the more remote secondary zone.

The tertiary zone is for seldom-used or large items. For example, locating printers and copiers outside your immediate scope of reach is ideal for several reasons. First, these larger items won't take up all the primary desktop space. Second, using them requires you to take an intentional microbreak.

Chairs

The founding fathers of the United States used the guiding principles of the Constitution as a foundation for success. Home builders know that they have to pour the concrete foundation first before they can do any other construction. As any teacher knows, reading provides the foundation for long-term academic success. Similarly, the office chair is the foundation of success for a properly set up workstation.

When you assess or set up your workstation, the chair that you choose goes a long way in determining your long-term success in staying symptom free. It is the single most important element and the foundation of the process. Each of the various types of chairs is correct for the specific type of job it was designed for. You cannot assume that the cushiony chair you have is correct for you because of the softness of the leather or the style of the backrest. When it comes to your chair, substance is everything over style.

Executive Chairs

An executive chair (figure 7.6) is often one piece. The seat pan, the part you sit on, and the backrest move as one unit. The chair may or may not have a height adjustment feature. The armrests usually are not removable and are fixed in height and shape. The chair will tilt in one piece, often with only a knob under the seat pan to regulate the tension that governs how easily the chair reclines when you lean back.

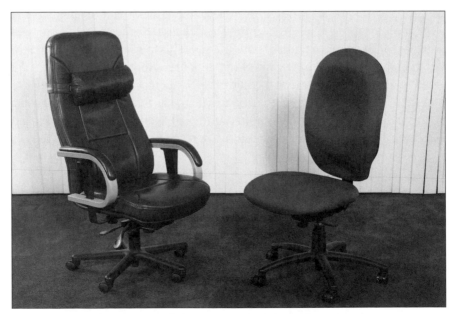

Figure 7.6 An executive chair (left) and a task chair (right).

The chair will not lock in an upright position. Typically there are no backrest height, depth, or tilt adjustments.

These chairs are best for meeting rooms where comfort and casual conversation are necessary. They offer an impression of style and comfort. If you hold meetings at your desk, these chairs are appropriate for your guests. They are appropriate for you when you are doing short-term writing or reviewing documents at your desk, dictating, using the phone extensively, and so on. The executive style chair is not appropriate for prolonged desk work or data entry jobs that require prolonged computer, 10-key, drafting, editing, or other types of task work. It's not that you can't type, write, review, or work in these chairs; they're simply not designed to provide you the necessary support or adjustments that you need over prolonged periods to be comfortable. These chairs can range in cost from a few hundred dollars to several thousand. Like everything, you get what you pay for.

Task Chairs

Task chairs (see figure 7.6) are the chairs used by most people for whom this chapter was written—those who spend hours at a time at home or at an office answering phones, planning meetings, entering data on the computer, using a 10-key pad, preparing legal documents, drafting letters, designing buildings and roads, reconciling invoices, preparing financial records, making marketing brochures, and writing manuscripts, among other tasks. A good task chair is the most important feature of any home or office workstation setup. A good task chair can make up for a poor overall arrangement, but a bad task chair can render thousands of dollars of furniture and ergonomic aides meaningless. The chair is, to some degree, both part of the problem and the solution. Addressing it is paramount.

A good task chair has several key features. First, it should be in two pieces, having the seat pan separate from the backrest. Each should have independent tilt adjustment, allowing you to maneuver either the seat pan or backrest independent of the other. Nearly all have an adjustable seat pan height. An adjustable backrest height is helpful as well. A locking mechanism should hold the chair in an upright, working position and be easy to unlock to allow reclining to a resting position.

Although armrests are thought to be mandatory in a good chair, this is incorrect. Armrests are not necessary and should be removable and adjustable. If the chair does have armrests, they should be low enough to slide under the keyboard surface when you push the chair forward. Adjustability is important.

A task chair may cost a hundred dollars to several thousand. When in doubt, spend a little extra on the chair. In the long run, you'll be thankful. After all, it is the foundation of your work area setup.

Getting a Good Fit

Chair dimensions are based on anthropometric tables, with adjustments designed to accommodate up to 95 percent of the general population. Standard height adjustments range from 16 to 21 inches (41 to 53 cm), and standard seat pan depths range from 15 to 19 inches (38 to 48 cm).

A fancy chair doesn't necessarily mean that you are in the clear. A chair loaded with all the contours and adjustments needed to be comfortable won't help if you don't know how to use them. Often a chair is simply in the work area when a new employee arrives and is used just as the last user left it. Do not assume the chair you inherit in a new work area is ready for your use.

Ask yourself whether your chair can be adjusted and, if so, whether are you using all the features that the chair has to offer. You can make a substantial improvement on your work comfort by making even small adjustments of the chair. Here are the main positional keys to getting a properly adjusted chair (table 7.2).

Table 7.2   Adjusting Your Workstation
Make the measurements and adjustments in order.

	Measurement	Adjustment	Notes
1. Chair height	While seated, measure from the floor to the back of the knee.	Add 1 inch (2.5 cm) to the measurement to determine the proper chair height.	The hips should be slightly higher than the knees.
2. Seat depth	While seated, measure from the buttock to the back of the knee.	Subtract 1 to 2 inches (2.5 to 5 cm) from the measurement to determine the proper seat depth.	There should be about a two-finger gap from the front edge of the chair to the lower leg.
3. Backrest height	While seated, measure from the seat pan to the bottom of the shoulder blade.	Add 2 inches (5 cm) to the measurement to determine the ideal backrest height.	The backrest should support at least to the shoulder blade. An open-back chair is best.
4. Armrest height (optional)	While seated, measure from the floor to the elbow while the elbow is bent 90 degrees.	Subtract 1 inch (2.5 cm) from the measurement to determine the proper armrest height.	Armrests should be lower than the level of the elbows.
5. Keyboard and mouse surface height	While seated, measure from the floor to the elbow while the elbow is bent 90 degrees.	Add 1 inch (2.5 cm) to the measurement to determine the proper keyboard and mouse surface height.	The forearms should be parallel to the floor when you are keying. The hands should float above the keys, not rest on the wrist pad. If resting, turn the hands in a thumbs-up position to relax the muscles. The mouse and keyboard should be on the same surface level, close together.
6. Desktop and writing surface	Measure from the floor to the desktop.	Optional, depending on preferences for the keyboard and mouse surface.	You may place the keyboard on a desktop or use a drop-down keyboard tray. A split desktop in which you have one height for keying and another height for writing is acceptable.
7. Monitor height and distance	While seated fully upright, measure from the floor to eye level.	The top line of text should be at eye level unless you wear bifocals. The monitor should be one arm's reach away.	If you wear bifocals, the top line of text should be 2 inches (5 cm) below eye level.

1. When you are seated, your thighs should slope slightly downward. That is, your hips should be slightly higher than your knees (figure 7.7). The distance from the back of your knee to the floor, say 17 inches (43 cm), should be slightly exceeded by the distance from the floor to the top of the seat pan, say 18 inches (46 cm). Often a slight forward tilt of the seat pan is useful to find a comfortable lower back position as well.

2. When you are seated, there should be a space of two finger widths from the front edge of the chair to the back of your knee. The distance from the back of your buttocks to the back of your knee, say 18 inches (46 cm), should be slightly greater that the distance from the back of the seat rest to the front edge

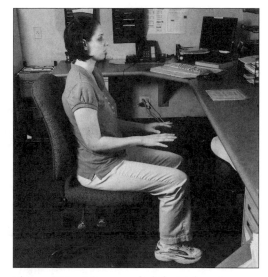

Figure 7.7   Hips are slightly higher than knees.

of the chair, say 17 inches (43 cm). Additionally, the edge of the seat pan should curve down slightly in what is called a waterfall design. This form relieves pressure on the back of the thighs where the sciatic nerve courses.

3. When you are seated at the proper chair height (18 inches [46 cm], for example), the backrest should come at least to a level just below the bottom of your shoulder blades. Often, the backrest is far too low, and the built-in lumbar support hits the occupant in the wallet (sacral) area. This is not correct. In most cases, the backrest should be raised all the way up so that the lower back support contacts you above the belt line, not at or below it. A backrest that is too low will push you forward in the chair, away from the support offered by the backrest. The result will be discomfort between your shoulder blades.

4. The backrest should be locked upright (figure 7.8a) so that when you lean back the chair does not recline (figure 7.8b). Often people like to use their task chairs to recline back to rest or work. This positioning is not correct. The backrest should be locked upright and tilted forward slightly so that the chair stays in contact with you in an upright position rather than your having to lean back to reach it.

5. When you are seated, the width of the chair should allow you room to let your hands touch the seat. You do not need any more room than that. Measure your width from buttock to buttock. If the chair gives you at least that plus an inch (2.5 cm), it will not be too small.

6. When you are seated at the proper height, hold out your hands as if to type (see figure 7.7). The forearms should be parallel to the floor, shoulders relaxed, and elbows resting comfortably at your sides. Measure the distance from the bottom of your elbow to the floor, 27 inches (69 cm), for example. This number tells you two things. First, the armrests need to be lower than that height (27 inches) measured from the floor to the top of the armrests. If they do not go lower than the undersurface of the desk or keyboard tray height, you need to remove them. Second, the floor-to-

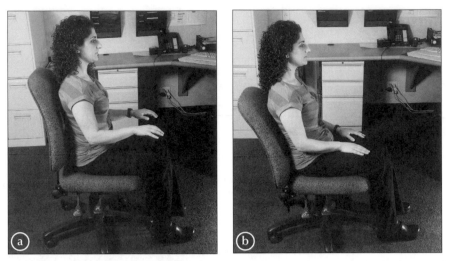

Figure 7.8 *(a)* In correct position, the backrest is locked upright and slightly tilted forward. *(b)* If the backrest isn't locked, the chair back will recline if you lean back, creating a poor working posture.

elbow number tells you the correct keyboard tray height, if typing is a primary job function, or the correct desktop height, if writing is a primary task. For example, for typing, the keyboard tray surface should be 27 inches from the floor. The general goal is to get your forearms parallel to the floor, wrists straight, and the keyboard or desktop at the same level as your forearms.

7. When you are seated, your eyes should be level with the top line of text shown on the monitor. For example, if the distance from the floor to the seat is 18 inches (46 cm) and the seat to your eyes is another 30 inches (76 cm), the top line of text when the monitor is placed on the desktop should be 48 inches (122 cm) from the floor. Finding the correct height for the monitor is not as hard as it may seem. You already know the desktop height (30 inches in our example), so simply measure the monitor from the stand to the top line of text. The numbers should add up to your starting measurement of 48 inches. You can use risers to add to the height of the monitor but cannot easily lower the height after the monitor is on the desk. In these cases, you will need to raise the chair and use a footrest to make the line of vision parallel to the floor. If you wear bifocals, the general rule is to subtract 2 inches (5 cm) from the monitor height. In our example, the proper monitor height would be 46 inches (117 cm) from the floor if the user wears bifocals.

Computer Equipment

The ideal height for the keyboard and mouse is determined by the floor-to-elbow height taken after the chair height is set properly, with the hips slightly higher than the knees. Avoid the error that many new users make by beginning work in the area just as the prior occupant left it. As legendary basketball coach John Wooden said, "If you don't have time to do it right, when will you have time to do it over?" Take the time to use these guidelines to set up your work area correctly from the start.

If your furniture is adjustable, you have many options. If not, you can use drop-down keyboard trays, monitor risers, and footrests to make necessary adjustments. Let's continue with the keyboard and mouse.

Your mouse and keyboard should always be on the same surface at the same level. Placing a keyboard on a drop-down tray and the mouse on the desktop is a prime cause of overreaching and will readily lead to shoulder tendinitis, tennis elbow, and other maladies.

Use an adjustable height keyboard tray only if your knees have room to slide in under it when you are working. If your desk is already too low, using a drop-down tray may not be advantageous because your knees may get in the way. In this case, you will have to place the keyboard and mouse on the desktop. If this positioning places your forearms not parallel to the floor, you will need to raise your chair and use a footrest to make up the distance so that your feet maintain a firm contact position. The keyboard should be tilted so that your wrists are straight, not cocked up (extended) or curled forward (flexed).

A well-designed keyboard tray has enough room for both the keyboard and mouse. Optimally, the tray will allow the mouse to be slightly forward and closer to you to negate further reaching. The articulating arm, the device that holds the keyboard tray to the undersurface of the desk, typically is 18 or 22 inches (46 to 56 cm) long. You will need to measure to verify that your keyboard tray will slide all the way back under the desk when you push it back. If you have a standard 22-inch tray, in some situations you will not be able to install it all the way back without the keyboard sticking out, so be sure to get the shorter 18-inch size. Just verify the placement before you start the installation so that you don't end up with the keyboard sticking out unnecessarily.

Floor Mats and Footrests

Floor mats are an excellent addition to a work area either at home or at an office. Consider the surface that you are putting them on, carpet or hard flooring. The bottom of the floor mat will vary depending on which type of surface you are buying it for. Generally, mats made for a low pile carpet or a no pile smooth-surface carpet work well. The floor mats need to cover only the area traversed by your chair as you move around in the work space, not the entire work area. People who have multiple work areas within their desk area, such as a writing surface, keying area, and meeting desk, benefit most from using a floor mat because it allows them to glide the chair about the area without having to pull themselves in the chair from one spot to another.

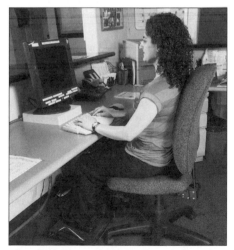

Figure 7.9   Use a footrest if your feet aren't firmly on the ground when you sit in a chair set to the proper height.

Pincher grip pulling is often a major cause for the onset of carpal tunnel issues.

A footrest (figure 7.9) is necessary if you cannot place your feet firmly on the ground. This issue occurs most often when the chair is high because the keyboard and mouse are on the desktop or because the monitor cannot be lowered. This situation happens if the height of your desk cannot be adjusted down or you are not able to use a drop-down keyboard tray because your knees hit it. A footrest allows you to maintain a parallel line of view to the top of the monitor, keep your forearms parallel to the floor while keying, and keep the hips slightly higher than the knees when the furniture is not fully adjustable or compatible to your dimensions.

Myth

I NEED ARMRESTS ON MY CHAIR AND A WRIST REST FOR MY KEYBOARD

Armrests are not necessary to have a properly set up workstation. Armrests are optional. In fact, most people who do desk and data entry work should remove armrests. Often armrests are too high, contributing to joint, nerve, and muscle-related problems.

If you use armrests, they should be lower than the bottom surface of the desktop or keyboard tray. Your chair should be able to slide fully under the desk or keyboard. Also, armrests should be lower than the height of your elbows when you sit in the chair and your arm is at your side. To use the armrests, you should have to lower your shoulder blade slightly or lean a little onto the armrests.

Wrist rests should be used for resting, not working. Unfortunately, rather than properly floating the hands over the keys, many users rest their wrists on the wrist rest while working. This practice leads to nerve compression problems, among others. If the keyboard is positioned at the proper height, no wrist rest is needed at all.

Wrist rests are appropriate if you use them properly. They should be no higher than the front edge of the keyboard and should be used only when resting, not typing. The best way to use those rests is to place your hands on them with your fifth finger down and thumb up. This position will help turn off the muscles of the upper neck, shoulder, and wrist extensors, which are commonly overworked in people who type a lot. When typing and keying, the proper technique is to float your hands across the keys and glide the mouse over the pad. Avoid the pivoting motion that occurs when you anchor the hands by resting them on the wrist rest. The same is true for armrests. You should not anchor your wrist on the mouse pad or keep your elbow and forearm stationary on the armrests. Doing so creates compression issues and the likelihood of nerve irritation. If the heights are correct and your forearms are parallel to the floor when in the keying and mousing positions, you should be able to float your hands across the keys. This position forces you to use the larger joints and muscles rather than the smaller ones that are easily irritated.

We discussed monitor height earlier. As for distance, the general rule is to place the monitor at least one arm's length away. For those with a deep corner in the work area, there is generally no problem. But many try to place the monitor on a standard height desktop that has a depth of only 24 or 28 inches (61 or 71 cm). Proper placement is difficult if the keyboard and mouse are also on the desktop because the desk may not be deep enough to accommodate all the items. In years past, this problem was more difficult to solve, but the widespread adoption of flat screen technology has made the issue much easier to remedy. If you don't have a flat screen, you may have to move your desk a few inches (5 to 10 cm) out away from the wall to fit the monitor on the desk. The money that you spend now to upgrade your equipment is minimal compared with the money that you will spend later on medical care if you experience symptoms. Flat screen monitors are priced now so usually they are not a major set-up expense.

The monitor may be tilted slightly up or down as comfort allows to negate glare from overhead lighting or a nearby window. A rule of thumb is to tilt the face of the monitor no more than 10 degrees up or down to resolve glare. You may want to use a glare hood if the tilt does not solve the problem.

The size of the mouse is important. Some are so small that you need to contort your hand as if you are cupping an egg just to use it. Others are so large that you can't easily use them. If you are comfortable using a trackball mouse, feel free to continue using it. But adjusting the heights and distances and using the correct technique is superior to switching to a trackball mouse. A vertical mouse should fit in your hand in a shape similar to the position you use just before shaking hands. A standard-shaped mouse should fit from the crease of your wrist to the tip of your middle finger.

Have a family member or coworker help you with some of the measurements. Another excellent way to assess your setup is to ask a friend to take digital photos from several angles. Analyze your positioning in regard to the height of your knees and hips, position of your wrists and forearms, line of view to the monitor, tilted angle of the chair back, and amount of forward reach to the keyboard and mouse. Then make some of the adjustments noted in this chapter.

THE FINISHING TOUCHES

In this chapter we have discussed the primary adjustments to make to your office or home computer workstation. Some of you likely already have an excellent setup and need only a small item here or there to enhance your comfort. This section is devoted to inexpensive products that you can use to ease strain or enhance your comfort while you work. Many companies carry these items, and you can view them easily on a plethora of websites. As a reference, we've provided one company contact that we particularly like if you have product questions.

Mouse Mate

Some people experience discomfort because the mouse is too small for their hand size. A mouse mate, which costs $15 or less, functionally enlarges the size of the mouse, making it fit in the palm more comfortably. Simple to use, the mouse mate comes with a small piece of Velcro that you attach to the back of the mouse. Then you simply attach the mouse mate to the Velcro to keep it in place. If another person uses the mouse, he or she can quickly remove the mouse mate. You'll be able to glide your hand more easily over the mouse surface, easing upper neck strain and hand-specific pain. Mouse mates work well and are an inexpensive way to change the size of your mouse without buying a new one.

Mouse Bridge

The mouse bridge, which costs $25 or less, helps ease neck and upper back discomfort by effectively bringing the mouse closer to the user. If you recall, one of our principle objectives is to place the mouse directly adjacent to the keyboard. When space for the mouse is not available, the mouse bridge allows you to put it directly on top of the keyboard, thereby minimizing forward reach. Remember that excessive forward reach is one of the three primary culprits that lead to neck and upper back discomfort. A small piece of thin plastic, the mouse bridge covers the numeric part on the right-hand aspect of the keyboard. If you don't use those right-hand numbers, the mouse bridge can offer a large benefit for a small price.

Vu-Ryte Document Holder

Computer users often have to input data or copy documents. In many workstations the keyboard tray serves as a platform for the paperwork, and the keyboard is an arm's reach away on the desktop. That arrangement is not the way to do it. Many document holders are simple easels that hold the papers off to the side of the monitor. The Vu-Ryte document holder, which costs $55 or less, aligns the paperwork directly in front of the monitor and in line with the keyboard, thereby lessening reach and avoiding the asymmetrical positioning created by most document holders. Recall that one of the three main ergonomic culprits that lead to spinal pain is an unbalanced or asymmetrically aligned work area. The Vu-Ryte document holder overcomes this problem and is fully adjustable so that those with space issues can find a way to fit it to the work area.

Mouse Cord Clips

Mouse cord clips, which cost about 15 cents each, are perhaps the best little discovery of all. These cord clips are really wax-backed paper holders that you would use to attach to your refrigerator or side of your desk. You can buy them at any office supply store. They come in packs of 12 or so and are intended to hold papers and small notes left lying around the house or office. The value is that they help keep the mouse cord in place, effectively stopping the migration of the mouse toward the back of the desk. Over time as you use the mouse, the weight of the mouse cord slowly pulls the mouse farther away from you as it hangs off the back of the desk. The clip negates the pull and allows you to position the mouse wherever you want it and keep it there. Give a little cord slack and place the cord clip somewhere near the back of the work area, out of the way. The clip is easily changeable, so don't worry about placing it in the wrong spot. You will notice that the mouse stays where you want it as opposed to creeping continually toward the back of your desk. A clip is well worth the investment.

CREATE YOUR IDEAL OFFICE

In this chapter we've explained that neck and lower back discomfort can be a function of a poor ergonomic setup. Understanding that symptoms occur over time as a result of repeated exposure is the first element of the chapter. Next, you can use the information to analyze your work area for the three most common setup errors—overreaching, incorrect heights, and an unbalanced work area—and then make adjustments to ease unwanted muscle and joint pain. By following the guidelines, beginning with the chair, you have at your disposal a powerful tool in your quest to feel better.

PART

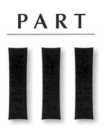

Working With Your Doctor

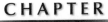

CHAPTER

8

Choosing a Doctor

D r. Joseph P. Van Der Muelen, the former president of the USC school of medicine once said, "A patient does not care how much you know until they know how much you care." This quote succinctly expresses our style of medicine: We care.

Thirty-two professions, from athletic trainers to neurosurgeons, are involved in spine care. How do you find a doctor to solve your spine problems, and how do you know that she or he is right for you? In a survey at Methodist Hospital in 2002, 144 patients with histories of moderate to severe spine pain, 55 of whom previously had surgery, were asked what they considered most important in choosing a doctor. The top three characteristics cited were someone whom they could trust and who cared, someone who was competent, and someone who was available. When doctors were asked the same question, most picked competence. What all patients want is someone with all these qualities. If your health care provider doesn't exhibit these qualities and fails to recognize a serious problem, the rest of your life could be significantly affected.

Consider John's story. John had been to six doctors about the pain that had kept him from working for 6 months. He had been treated with opioid medication, physical therapy, and acupuncture. Then he was told that he needed surgery. One consultant suggested that he seek psychological help. Finally, his last doctor took a thorough history and performed a complete examination in which the doctor asked John to remove his shirt. Was it important for John to take off his shirt? Yes. John's skin showed the scars of a case of shingles. John was prescribed a simple pain-modulating drug to stop nerve pain (neuralgia), which is caused by shingles. Two weeks later, John was back to work.

If John's prior doctors had just examined his skin, he may have been properly treated sooner. Prescriptions from narcotics to surgery had been given with good intentions but were ill advised because an adequate history was not taken and a thorough physical examination was not performed. Patients who are not asked for their thorough history, are not given a complete physical exam, or are subjected to hastily ordered tests and medication often are misdiagnosed or mistreated. They get caught in the web of spine pain specialists, from neurosurgeons to massage therapists. Patients may undergo a series of hastily ordered and unnecessary tests, muscular and spinal injections, indwelling narcotic pumps, manipulations, spinal traction gadgets, therapies, and even surgery.

This chapter will assist you in picking a health care professional, one who is competent, empathic, and available. You need not go down the road that John did.

EXPECTATIONS AND REALITY

What should you expect from your health care professional? Does the fact that the person has a sign on the door or letters after his or her name indicate that he or she is competent? Understanding the reality of the medical world today can help you realize what is going on and avoid what happened to John.

Since the 1950s we have gained more medical knowledge than we did in the preceding 2,000 years. With that has come a meteoric rise in the number of health care professionals, technological advances that spawned tests such as CT scans and MRIs, invasive medical interventions such as spinal blocks and injections of all sorts, and numerous medications. Noninvasive interventions such as physical therapy, chiropractic, traction, heat, and acupuncture have ballooned as well. Devices such as TENS units, biofeedback, and a full arsenal of FDA-approved medications and nonapproved holistic remedies have been prescribed. Is it possible that each of the many diverse and sometimes contradictory treatments work for every type of back pain? Of course not. However each particular type of spine pain has its own particular remedy.

When you look at all these treatments, examine your health care provider's credentials, and recognize possible conflicts of interest, you begin to realize the stew that you can get yourself into if your health care professional cannot back up the sign over the door or the letters following her or his name. Some of these treatments will do no harm, but many can and do.

Since 1950 spine care cost has increased 40-fold. This increase is not because of doctor costs. Instead, 95 percent of this increase is because of testing and treatment. Over the last 50 years, the cost of neck and back care in the United States has risen 22 times the rate of inflation. Neck and lumbosacral spinal problems have created a $110 billion business.

The competition to cure your back problem is fast and furious. On one side, it is led by the businesses that lose $80 billion each year through workers compensation claims and to insurance companies. On the other side, a slew of professionals, and some who are not so professional, try to earn or take those billions. The effect on all Americans in a global economy is a diminished ability to compete because similar populations in Asia and India pay far less in medical costs.

You must choose a spine care specialist whom you can trust with your health. The problem is not that we have too many choices of health care professionals, diagnostic tests, and treatments, both invasive and noninvasive. Instead, the issue concerns making the right choice for your particular problem. An accurate diagnosis is key.

In our experience, however, many patients choose their doctors as they might pick a head of lettuce at a grocery store. They listen to the suggestion of a recent acquaintance as if it came from someone with years of training.

Myth

MY DOCTOR WILL KNOW WHAT'S WRONG

Your doctor will not be able to identify the problem without your help. An accurate diagnosis requires a detailed history. Your doctor does not have a crystal ball, and he or she most likely wasn't there when your discomfort started.

Often patients get upset with doctors because doctors ask too many questions during an initial consultation. As the patient, you need to be prepared to give an accurate and detailed history regarding your symptoms. Approximations are fine in terms of dates, but you need to be specific concerning the symptoms: When does it hurt? Where does it hurt? What does the hurt feel like? How long has it been this way? What makes you feel better? What makes you feel worse? What is the overall trend of the discomfort (is it getting better, worse, or not changing)?

Although most conditions are not severe, particular warning signs may indicate that your condition is far more complicated than musculoskeletal spinal pain. For example, your doctor needs to know whether your pain has coincided with a fever, recent illness, dental visit, or other medical procedure. For neck and upper torso discomfort, have you had a persistent or hacking cough? Do symptoms increase with exertion? Is neck stiffness associated with headaches and a high fever? In the lumbar area, does the discomfort worsen after a meal? Does it worsen when you urinate or empty the bowel? Is a discoloration or warm area present over the spine or adjacent hip? These are all relevant bits of information that your doctor needs to know.

Your doctor also has to take the time to do a thorough examination. In doing so, she or he is relying on you to provide accurate responses. For example, does a test hurt because the doctor is grabbing your leg too hard or because the test reproduces your symptoms? If you are having difficulty grasping a cup, is it because your hand is weak or because it hurts? Your response is important. Your doctor doesn't know unless you speak up.

Without gathering a complete history, fully examining the area, ordering the proper lab tests, and providing the necessary prescription, whether medication, therapy, or specialist intervention, your physician cannot fully help you. Ultimately, the success of your doctor visit lies as much with you as with your physician.

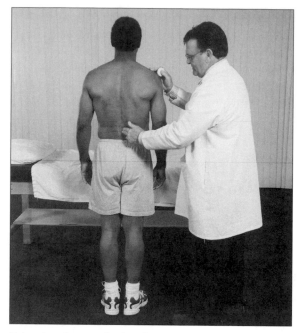

Take the time to find a doctor you can trust.

You must pay as much attention to choosing who is going to be in charge of your treatment as you do when picking a school for your child. Take time to investigate before choosing a health care professional or a therapist. Don't simply ask a friend whom she or he uses. Make it your responsibility. Remember that the right diagnosis and treatment are not possible without an accurate and detailed history, a thorough physical examination, and the right diagnostician.

What went wrong in John's case? It could have been that John was a bad historian who was reluctant to tell the doctor everything. It could have been that the health care professionals whom he saw were in a rush. It could have been that the health care professionals whom he saw were inadequately trained or that John's problem was beyond their competency. It could have been that John didn't receive an adequate exam. It could have been one of these things, some of them, or all of them. In John's case a proper diagnosis was made possible because the health care professional simply asked John to take off his shirt and noticed the infection under his skin.

EVALUATING YOUR HEALTH CARE PROFESSIONAL

First, you need to ask yourself what you prefer. Second, you need to learn how to assess the ability of your health care professional.

Before choosing a health care professional, some people ask friends for recommendations, check the physician's credentials, or call the local hospital for a referral. In this age of managed care, you also need to check the list of doctors who will accept your insurance provider. None of these methods are foolproof in identifying a qualified professional with whom you feel comfortable to share your innermost feelings and concerns about your back and neck problems.

Perhaps one of the most important steps to take when selecting a physician to diagnose and treat a spinal problem is to know yourself, including your personal likes and dislikes. As you choose a physician, consider these 20 questions. Some of the questions pertain to your initial selection of a physician. Others are to consider after you've seen this physician several times to help you make sure that you have chosen the right doctor for you.

Choosing a Physician: 20 Questions

1. Would you feel more comfortable with a man or woman?

2. Should the physician be older than you, the same age, or younger?

3. Do you have a preference about educational background?

4. Is the doctor board certified, that is, has the doctor passed a standard exam given by the governing board in his or her specialty?

5. Where did the doctor go to medical school? Your local medical society can provide this information or look online at www.docboard.org/docfinder.html.

6. Is the doctor involved in any academic pursuits, such as teaching, writing, or research? A doctor who teaches, writes, or conducts research may be more up to date in the latest developments in the field.

7. Where does the doctor have hospital privileges, and where are those hospitals located? Some doctors may not admit patients to certain hospitals, and this can be an important consideration for older adults with health problems.

8. Does the doctor accept your health insurance, or is the doctor a member of the medical panel associated with your HMO?

9. Is the doctor's staff friendly and reassuring? Do they smile and make you feel valued? Chances are that the staff reflects the personality of the physician.

10. What are the doctor's office hours? Are these hours convenient for you or the person who is transporting you?

11. During the initial visit, does the doctor conduct a thorough review of your medical history, including medications, past surgery, lifestyle habits, and family history?

12. Does the doctor look at you when greeting you, as though you are a person of value?

13. How much time does the doctor spend on follow-up visits?

14. Does the doctor examine you thoroughly and perform a complete spine exam?

15. Does the doctor order tests readily, or does she or he tend to minimize your concerns?

16. Is the doctor ready to give you a prescription without explaining more about the side effects?

17. Does the doctor return your phone calls?

18. Does the doctor make you feel that your health comes above all else? Alternatively, do you fear that your health care plan dictates the quality of care that you receive?

19. If you need hospitalization, will this doctor still treat you, or will you be delegated to a specialist at the hospital who knows nothing about you as a person? You must ask your doctor this question.

20. Does the doctor use specialists to assist in your situation if you request one? (Sometimes health plans discourage physicians from referring to other specialists,

or the physician may have bad rapport with other specialists. Both are warning signs to find a new physician or get a new health plan.)

When you are seeing a specialist, make sure that you bring all your studies—MRI, CT—and laboratory data. When the history and physical exam are over, ask the doctor to identify exactly what structure he or she believes is causing your pain. If the doctor cannot do this, it is a red flag.

YOU HAVE THE POWER

Seek a spine specialist who has a reputation for excellent bedside manner—one who talks to you, not at you. If you are referred to a pain specialist, check her or his credentials carefully. Not all pain specialists are of equal competence. Almost anyone can claim to treat pain, but few are specifically trained in this specialty. Call your local hospital or ask ER nurses or your doctor whom they see or would see if they had your problem.

If you need a surgeon, find one with an impressive record in treating spine problems like yours. If you have been prescribed opioid medications or injections, do not be afraid to ask for a second opinion. Any physician who is confident of her or his diagnosis or treatment plan will welcome this.

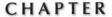

CHAPTER

Getting the
Right Diagnosis

S t. Peter's Cathedral, the Coliseum in Rome, the Eiffel Tower, the Blue Mosque in Turkey, and the pyramids are incredible achievements of architectural genius that have endured for centuries. Their awesome structures support the beams of the towers, the vaults, and all the tons of masonry needed in each of these wonders of the world.

The human body is likewise marvelous. The skeleton, with the spine being its main component, is the amazing structure that supports the body. Through the spine runs all the circuitry of the spinal cord and its roots. But the body is not a static structure to be visited and looked at. The body is able to lift, bend, twist, run, and jump. The body is a wonder of the world in motion.

What does this analogy mean to back and neck disorders and your quest to find the right diagnosis and treatment? Your health care professional must be able to examine your structure and assess what is wrong and why so that any treatment applied will help you, not harm you. He or she does this by obtaining a complete medical history and thoroughly examining your body. From the information gathered through these methods, he or she can prescribe the treatment to help you.

A health care professional's education, training, and experience will help her or him make this diagnosis, but the diagnosis will be accurate only if the patient provides an adequate history and the health care professional performs an adequate exam. You and your health care professional are a team.

Some doctors and patients sometimes question the necessity of obtaining a detailed history or conducting a physical exam in light of the technological advances in body scans and other diagnostic tests. Technological advances have changed what we know of the body. But technology is a double-edged sword. Often it leads to a wrong conclusion, and wrong conclusions lead to useless treatment that may make back and neck problems worse or even cause permanent injury.

TECHNOLOGY AND THE CLINICIAN

In the 1970s and 1980s, CT scans and MRI scans took the mystery out of the spine's structure and identified narrowing of the facettes, degenerative arthritis, narrowing of the canals, and even spinal tumors. The treatment modalities for spinal pain exploded. Just as cell phones have made telegrams and phone booths obsolete, so the new scan technology led many health care professionals to believe that a history and physical exam were not needed. Because these scans can identify abnormalities in the spinal structure, you would think that specific treatments could be rendered to fix them. The use of braces, spinal injections, manipulations, and traction devices increased, but studies showed little improvement and, in fact, worse results in some cases. For instance, the number of people returning to work after injuries in the 1980s and 1990s decreased instead of increased. Dependence on these new technologies led us down the wrong path, confusing rather than clarifying diagnoses. Working hours lost because of spine pain soared during the 1980s and 1990s, the heyday of new technology. In many cases, technological advances made patients believe that their pain was worse than it really was.

In 1982 the journal *Spine* published an award-winning study showing that our revolutionary technology was not as effective as previously thought. Rather than enhancing accuracy for specific diagnoses, it often did the opposite. In the study, a radiologist diagnosed significant disease in half of a group of patients over age 50 who had no complaints of pain. Even patients 25 years old were diagnosed with significant spinal changes in 20 percent of cases. Those with no complaints were being diagnosed as having serious problems where none existed. The study showed that our reliance on these diagnostic tests led to misdiagnoses. Prescriptions based on misdiagnoses may lead to injury.

Furthermore, the study in *Spine* demonstrated the factors that determined whether surgery would be successful. Later, other studies showed that 86 percent of spinal surgeries were successful if the scan coincided with the history and physical exam, but only 36 percent of surgeries were favorable if the scan did not confirm the history and the physical exam. You would expect 33 percent for a placebo effect. In other words, if the scan did not support the history and the physical exam, the chances of a good outcome were no better than doing nothing, and in many cases, were much worse.

As we age, our spines naturally change. What is normal for a 20-year-old spine is not normal for a 60-year-old spine. Doctors treat symptoms, not scans. Several studies have confirmed that 50 percent of patients over 50 years old show some kind of abnormality on scans despite no symptoms. The body adapts to the anatomical changes from aging, for example, nerves move or flatten. An abnormal scan does not mean you have symptoms or even will develop them. In fact in 70 percent of those over 50, and in 90 percent of those over 70, it is common for multiple abnormalities to show up on a CT or MRI scan. Be sure your symptoms correspond to your scans.

HELP FOR A CORRECT DIAGNOSIS

To get a proper solution to your problem, you need a correct diagnosis. To do this, you and your doctor need HELP (history, exam, lab tests, prescription). A successful outcome to surgical treatment when a certain diagnosis is established occurs in 86 percent of cases versus a 36 percent success rate when the diagnosis is uncertain. By following the HELP method your doctor can arrive at a correct diagnosis. The history, physical exam, and laboratory tests—CT, MRI scan, EMG—lead to a proper prescription for your pain. If the first three elements do not support one another, a correct diagnosis is missed and the results of treatment may be abysmal and harmful. These three elements—history, physical exam, and lab results—must fit and support one to lead to a certain diagnosis of your spinal pain.

If your health care professional obtains a detailed history, does a thorough physical exam, orders the proper lab tests, and finds that these lab tests agree with the diagnosis made from the history and exam, the treatment prescription can be instituted and the likelihood of your having a good outcome is high (figure 9.1*a*). For example, if the history is supported by the exam and the labs show a lesion, herniated disc, or arthritic joint where the history and exam indicate, you can be confident that you have the correct diagnosis and the correct prescription can be given to help you. If the history, physical exam, and lab tests don't agree or localize the problem, the outcome is likely to be poor (figure 9.1*b*).

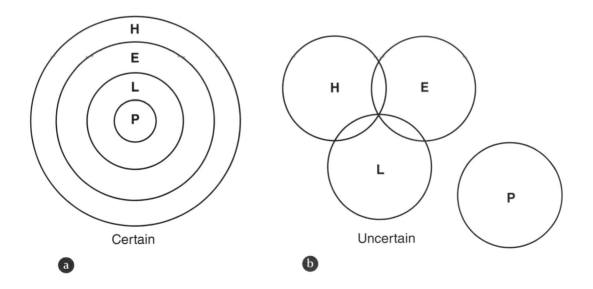

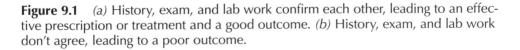

Figure 9.1 *(a)* History, exam, and lab work confirm each other, leading to an effective prescription or treatment and a good outcome. *(b)* History, exam, and lab work don't agree, leading to a poor outcome.

Therefore, making a diagnosis with CT and MRI scans by themselves can be dangerous to you, particularly if the EMG does not support them. If your medical professional relies only on a CT or MRI, you have better than a 50 percent chance of being misdiagnosed. A diagnosis made without a proper history and physical examination can lead to unnecessary interventions and a poor outcome.

Physicians are under serious time constraints today, enmeshed in what is called the time deficiency syndrome. They are required to review more tests and do more documentation in less time. Therefore, they have limited time to see patients. Several studies have shown that time is a crucial element in a proper diagnosis. When you have a problem, be sure to give your physician sufficient time to identify the problem. Often a patient will visit a doctor for another reason, a respiratory infection, for example, and mention an aching back just before leaving the appointment. Without time to do the proper history and physical examination, many health care professionals use the shotgun approach, ordering laboratory tests such as an X-ray or sending the patient to a therapist without any knowledge of the real problem. Don't expect good health care if you cannot give the doctor a good history and the time to take a proper history and physical examination.

The primary ethical principle for health care professionals is to do no harm. As a patient, you should know what a proper history and a physical exam entail and when to ask for a second opinion so that no harm comes to you.

Remember that most health care professionals are gatekeepers. They triage and identify problems. Back pain in the lumbosacral area may come from the spinal structure, a kidney infection, or problems of the bowel, rectum, testicle, or ovary. After your primary health care professional does an in-depth exam, he or she will determine whether you need further investigation by a spine specialist.

History

Dr. William Osler, a famous diagnostician, once said, "A patient who cannot give a good history and a doctor who cannot take one is in danger of giving and getting poor treatment." Be prepared to share your medical history with your health care provider.

The history of your back pain is like any other history: It has a beginning and an end. Before you go in to see the health care professional, write down your timetable. Dates don't have to be exact; approximations are fine. It may help to review your symptoms on a table like that shown in table 9.1 or fill out a patient history questionnaire like the one shown in figure 9.2. To fill out table 9.1, ask yourself what effect these items have on your symptoms.

Table 9.1 Review of Symptoms

	Better	Worse	Unchanged
Coughing or sneezing			
Straining			
Sitting			
Driving			
Bending forward			
Lying flat on back			
Lying flat on front			
Lying on right side			
Lying on left side			
Walking one block			
Walking two or three blocks			
Walking four to six blocks			
Walking more than six blocks			
Standing			
Twisting			
Twisting and bending forward			
Lifting			
Morning pain			
Day pain			
Night pain			
Working overhead			
Stiffness in morning			
Weather			
Menstrual			

Patient History

Chief complaint today (neck and right arm, back, back and left leg, midback, and so on)

_____

_____

When did the symptoms originally begin?

Neck and arms _____   Back and legs _____   Midback _____

Did your pain develop gradually or start suddenly? _____

Was it because of an injury? _____ If so, how did the injury occur? If both the neck and back are injured, please be specific as to how many injuries occurred and when.

_____

_____

_____

Are your symptoms now worse, better, or unchanged? _____

What is the ratio of your neck pain to your arm pain? (for example, 100% neck/0% arm) (How much more does your neck hurt than your arm?)

100/0	90/10	80/20	70/30	60/40	50/50
40/60	30/70	20/80	10/90	0/100	

What is the ratio of your back pain to your leg pain? (for example, 100% back/0% leg) (How much more does your back hurt than your leg?)

100/0	90/10	80/20	70/30	60/40	50/50
40/60	30/70	20/80	10/90	0/100	

Do you have numbness in your upper extremities? _____ yes _____ no

If yes, where? (neck, right arm, left arm, hand, fingers, etc.) _____

_____

_____

Do you have numbness in your lower extremities? _____ yes _____ no

If yes, where? (upper back, mid back, right leg, left leg, thigh, foot, and so on) _____

_____

_____

Do you have weakness in your upper extremities? _____ yes _____ no

If yes, where? (neck, right arm, left arm, hand, fingers, and so on) _____

_____

Figure 9.2 Patient history questionnaire.

Do you have weakness in your lower extremities? _____ yes _____ no

If yes, where? (upper back, mid back, right leg, left leg, thigh, foot, and so on) _____
What action is limited? _____
_____

Do you have bowel or bladder problems?

_____ none _____ incontinence _____ constipation _____ hesitancy _____ dribbling
_____ frequency

Rate the pain in your neck and arms on a scale of 1 to 10, 10 being the worst pain. _____

Rate the pain in your back and legs on a scale of 1 to 10, 10 being the worst pain. _____

What past treatments have made your neck and arm pain better? (ice, medication, physical therapy, acupuncture, and so on) _____
_____

What past treatments have made your back and leg pain better? (ice, medication, physical therapy, acupuncture, and so on) _____
_____

What past treatments have made your neck and arm pain worse? (ice, medication, physical therapy, acupuncture, and so on)_____
_____

What past treatments have made your back and leg pain worse? (ice, medication, physical therapy, acupuncture, and so on) _____
_____

What diagnostic studies have you had to your neck and arms (i.e., MRI, CT scan, myelogram, EMG or NCV, contrast CT, bone scan, discogram, tomogram)? Note the dates when you had these tests. If you have not had studies, please write "none." _____
_____
_____
_____

Have you had spinal surgery? _____ yes _____ no

If yes, when was the surgery performed? _____

Where was the surgery performed?_____

Who performed the surgery? _____

Did you experience a pain-free interval after surgery? _____ yes _____ no

If yes, how long were you pain free after surgery? _____

Figure 9.2, *continued*

Onset, Location, Radiation, and Type

Be prepared to tell the doctor about the onset, location, radiation, and type of pain. For instance, did the pain develop gradually or did it suddenly appear? Is the pain aching or stabbing? Where is it localized? As best as you can, identify the location of the pain with one finger. If the pain is more diffuse, tell your doctor. Does it radiate, and if so, does it radiate down the back of the leg or arm, the side, or the front? Does it go below the knee or elbow?

A health care professional should always have you fill out a pain diagram (figure 9.3). The pain diagram shows location, radiation, and type of pain. A picture sometimes is worth a thousand words. Take a completed copy of this diagram to your doctor.

Be prepared to tell your doctor what provokes the pain or makes it worse. By provoked, we mean the things or actions that cause the pain. For instance, with nerve pain, bending, lifting, twisting, and reaching bring on the pain. By worsening, we mean that when the pain is present, what makes it worse?

Be prepared to say what makes the pain better, either easing the pain or getting rid of it all together. Often people say that rest, lying down on the side, medication, traction, physical therapy, or epidurals help.

Be prepared to tell the health care professional about the duration of the pain. One patient said that she had horrific, sharp pain in her neck that simply paralyzed her. When asked chronologically when this happened and how long it lasted, she revealed that it happened one week earlier and lasted only a second or two. When the pain hit, she thought that she could do nothing but just stand there until it passed, which took only a second.

Make sure that you tell the doctor the quality of the pain, not only if it is a deep or dull ache but also if it's present all the time, worse in the morning, better at night, or worse when you turn, bend, lift, reach, or twist.

Associated Symptoms

Often symptoms are associated with the pain. These symptoms are probably the most important symptoms of all in determining the severity or urgency of a problem. Remember the voices of the spine. Here we can differentiate a good health care professional from one who may be beyond her or his competency. Your health care professional must always be ready to ask certain questions that tell her or him whether your problem is serious or not.

First, are there any new difficulties with urination or with bowel movements? New means since the onset of the symptoms. Second, is there any numbness, loss of sensation, increase in sensation as pins and needles or burning, or dysesthesia, a tingling or burning caused when that area of the skin is touched? Third, is any weakness present? This item may seem simple, but weakness comes in many forms. Some patients quickly answer yes, they have weakness, but when asked where, say they just can't get moving until they have breakfast. Be prepared to be specific. For example, you could say, "I can't use my right leg to go upstairs or get out of a chair." Weakness can also be assessed by how far you can walk or, if you go to a gym, the amount of weight that you can no longer tolerate during a particular exercise.

Pain Location, Radiation, Quantity, and Quality

Name _____ Age _____ Date _____

Where is your pain now? On the illustrations, marks the areas of your body where you feel active pain, numbness, pins and needles, or burning using the appropriate symbols. Mark areas of radiating pain using the appropriate symbol. Include all affected areas.

Active pain	Numbness	Pins and needles	Burning	Radiating pain
^^^^^	OOOOO	+++++	XXXXX	/////

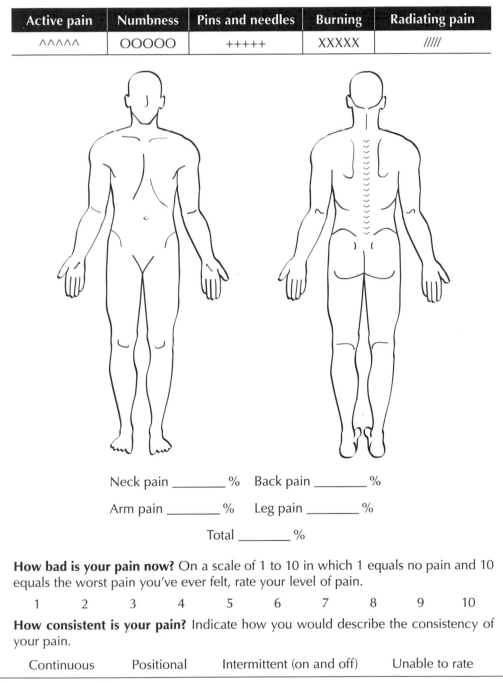

Neck pain _____ %   Back pain _____ %

Arm pain _____ %   Leg pain _____ %

Total _____ %

How bad is your pain now? On a scale of 1 to 10 in which 1 equals no pain and 10 equals the worst pain you've ever felt, rate your level of pain.

1   2   3   4   5   6   7   8   9   10

How consistent is your pain? Indicate how you would describe the consistency of your pain.

Continuous   Positional   Intermittent (on and off)   Unable to rate

Figure 9.3 Pain diagram.

Answering that you have weakness without a good explanation as to how it fits time wise with your symptoms can cause the health care professional to order unnecessary tests or put you through procedures that you may not need. If you can't tell exactly what muscle is weak, tell your doctor the action that you have difficulty performing. Is the weakness because of pain, or is the weakness unaccompanied by discomfort? Make certain that you tell your doctor when the weakness started. Be specific. If you think the doctor does not have time, ask for another appointment when he or she does.

Be prepared to tell the doctor of any bowel, bladder, or sexual changes associated with the pain problem. Make sure to tell your doctor whether the condition is preexisting. For example, men over 50 often have trouble urinating because of their prostates. For women, loss of urine or straining could be stress incontinence, which is often seen in older women or those who have had multiple children.

Be prepared to tell your doctor of any sensory loss or increased sensation. Remember that the sensation change is not pain, but a change in how you feel. Is the sensation decreased or increased compared with the uninvolved side? Sensory changes are often described as tingling, pins and needles, or burning. Total lack of sensation can occur, but initial nerve irritation is often associated with tingling.

Physical Examination

In a survey of patient satisfaction, patients noted that the two most important factors were whether the doctor showed concern and whether the patient believed that the doctor did an adequate examination. The last time you saw your doctor, were you satisfied with the examination?

In this section, we will look at what goes into a satisfactory initial examination for the evaluation of back and neck pain. You may wonder, shouldn't the health care professional know what to do? The problem is that the many types of health care professionals have different levels of competence in the field of back and neck pain. General practitioners, neurosurgeons, rheumatologists, urologists, gynecologists, chiropractors, physical therapists, exercise physiologists, neurologists, and spinal surgeons have different training and specialties. Pain specialists are often anesthesiologists. But whatever their training or specialty, the physical examination should be the same. Without this examination, their training means little.

If a proper examination is not performed, an accurate diagnosis probably will be missed, resulting in needed tests not being performed or needless tests being done. Your spine pain may not be properly treated, causing you harm by prolonging your pain or allowing your condition to become more serious. Medicine is a serious business. If something goes wrong, the patient pays for it, often both monetarily and physically. Be knowledgeable about what goes into an adequate examination. This knowledge enables you to demand more testing or treatment or ask for a second opinion, if you think it prudent. A good health care professional is never offended by such a request.

Remember that even a well-qualified physician cannot do an adequate exam if sufficient time isn't available. Be prepared to help the health care professional obtain a good history.

The physical exam consists of

- inspection,
- palpation,
- maneuvers (M), and
- a neurological examination (NE).

The neurological exam is complex and consists of motor, sensory, reflex, and gait evaluation. A mnemonic I use is nip'm (neurological exam, inspection, palpation, maneuvers), as in "nip 'em in the bud." A good exam nips the back or neck problem before it gets out of hand. The exam gives the doctor proof or confirms his or her suspicions. We will start with the *I* in nip'm and end with the *N* because the neurological exam is the most complicated.

Inspection

During the inspection, the doctor observes your body, especially the problem areas. Unfortunately, as in John's case, this part of the nip'm exam is sometimes overlooked. The inspection requires the patient to undress, which takes time and is sometimes inconvenient, especially if you are in the doctor's consultation room instead of the exam room. Time is of the essence for the health care professional, but the inspection is key to a proper diagnosis.

The doctor should observe the spine for asymmetry. Does the left side look like the right side? Is loss of muscle mass, or atrophy, evident in one muscle? This is a sign of a severe nerve injury. In one case, the patient had experienced numbness in his right hand. When it was examined, the hand showed atrophy in part of the muscle in his hand. This showed a serious problem, and he was advised to seek help immediately.

Is the spine straight or curved like an S (scoliosis), or is the patient bent over (kyphotic)? Is normal lordosis, the curve in the back and neck, present?

Inspection of the skin is one of the most important parts of the spine exam and the one most often overlooked. Is the skin normal, or are there signs of infection, a red hot area, or moles with darkened invading edges (melanoma), a malignant tumor?

Inspection alone can give the health care professional clues to the diagnosis. Often it opens up the differential diagnosis to include laboratory tests or skin biopsy, which can aid in treatment and may save your life. Birthmarks are of high significance because they can identify bone and nerve problems elsewhere. For example, neurofibroma is a soft mole associated with tumors on or near nerves in the brain or spine. Cafe au lait spots, light brown spots, also are associated with neurological problems elsewhere. Be sure to point out these birthmarks to your health care professional.

Palpation

Palpation is the hands-on touching of the back and related areas. Your participation in palpation is crucial. Identify to the doctor the areas that he or she is touching that are particularly painful and define the type of pain. Palpating a muscle next to the spinous process may give a deep, dull ache. Palpating a muscle over a spinous process where it is fractured, has a tumor, or is infected might cause excruciating pain.

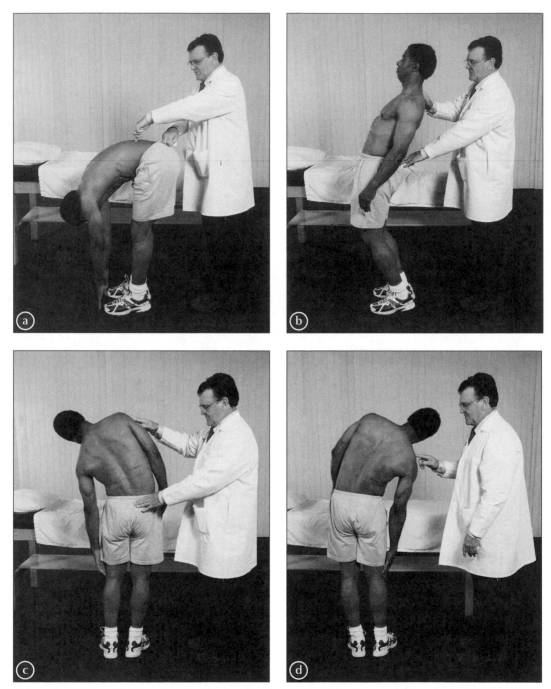

Figure 9.4 Range of motion for the low back: *(a)* flexion, *(b)* extension, *(c)* lateral bending to the left, *(d)* lateral bending to the right.

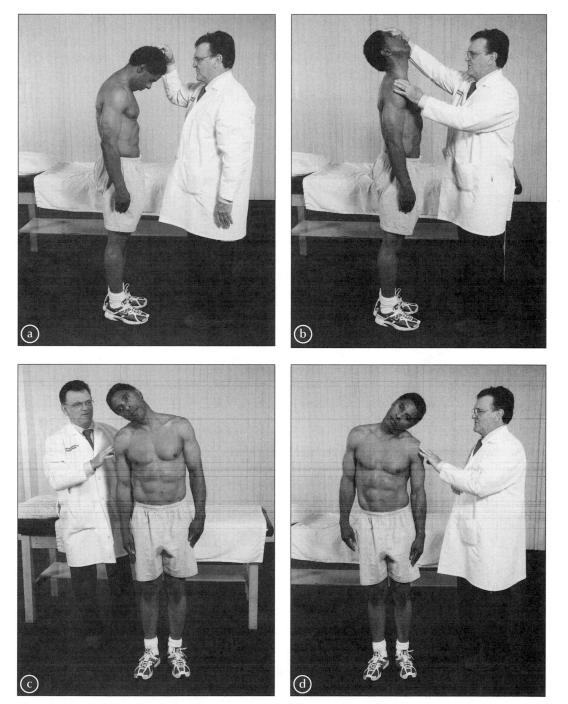

Figure 9.5 Range of motion for the neck: *(a)* flexion, *(b)* extension, *(c)* lateral bending to the right, *(d)* lateral bending to the left.

Maneuvers

This part of the exam is essential. A maneuver that reproduces your pain tells your doctor what part of your spine—nerve, muscle, or facette—is the culprit. Maneuvers include range of motion (ROM) of the low back (figure 9.4) and neck (figure 9.5), articulation or joint evaluation, and nerve stretch tests.

Only with your participation can the health care professional know what maneuvers cause the pain and exactly where in that maneuver the pain is provoked. Patient participation is as important in a spine examination as it is in an eye examination by an optometrist or ophthalmologist. If you don't tell the ophthalmologist which lens improves your vision, it is almost impossible for her or him to make the proper lenses for you.

ROM testing tells the health care professional whether your spinal motion is limited and in what positions. Together with inspection and palpation, this evaluation helps localize the area of involvement and at times helps the health care professional determine the underlying culprit of the pain.

In ROM testing, patient participation is critical. Tell the doctor when a particular motion causes pain and where that pain radiates. Sometimes ROM testing may cause numbness or tingling. Noting exactly what part of the arm, leg, hand, or foot tingles can identify the exact cause and location of the problem. Only you can provide your health care professional with this information. He or she may judge that a certain maneuver causes pain by your grimace but will not know that it causes tingling unless you say so. If your health care professional does not ask, be sure that you are prepared to tell him or her.

Joint and nerve stretch tests may be the most important in the diagnosis and localization of back and neck pain. They can identify the underlying structure that is injured and reproduce the voice of pain that you have, sometimes even reproducing the abnormal sensation or tingling. As in ROM testing, your verbal participation is essential. Remember that a nerve or joint cannot speak; it needs your interpretation. From there, the health care professional can make the diagnosis. Also, maneuvers can help the physician pick up adaptive shortening syndrome, the precursor of more serious problems, such as arthritis, caused by shortening.

We will cover the basic maneuvers every health care professional should perform. Specialists use other maneuvers that can be found in *Orthopedic Clinical Examination* by Joshua Cleland. We will divide the maneuvers covered here into low back and neck maneuvers.

The main spinal structures tested in the lower spine are

1. the sciatic nerve, through a straight leg raise test and flip test;
2. the hip joint, with the FABER, or Patrick, test;
3. the piriformis muscle, with the PECK test or abduction test; and
4. the femoral nerves, with the femoral stretch test.

The maneuvers for the neck are the Spurling test and the Bikele maneuver. Many other maneuvers are used in the back and neck. At a minimum, the straight leg test and the FABER test should be performed by your health care professional, whatever her or his expertise. The low back maneuvers are summarized in table 9.2.

Table 9.2   Low Back Maneuvers

	Maneuver	Sign of positive test	Location
Straight leg raise test	Lie on back with legs straight. The doctor lifts one straight leg to a 90-degree angle, if possible.	Test reproduces sharp, electric leg pain.	Nerve root in the back (sciatica)
FABER test	Lie on back. Bend one leg, placing heel on other knee. Turn bent leg out.	Leg shows limited motion. Test causes hip pain.	Hip joint
Femoral stretch test	Lie face down. The doctor lifts one thigh.	Pain in the groin or front of the thigh.	Femoral nerve in the groin
PECK test	As you sit, the doctor places his or her hands outside your knees. Push against the doctor's hands as the doctor resists.	Provokes pain in the buttocks or back.	Piriformis muscle as the nerve goes through or past it

Low Back Maneuvers

Straight Leg Raise Test

Lie down on your back. The health care professional will lift one of your legs (figure 9.6). Help your health care professional keep your leg straight at the knee and don't bend your knee as he or she lifts your leg. The other leg remains straight on the table. As your health care professional slowly lifts your leg, the nerve will stretch all the way from the nerve root to the foot. At about a 50- to 60-degree angle from the table, the nerve itself will move as it exits the vertebral canal through the foramen, where the nerve root lies and where most low back pathology occurs. When the leg is as high as it can go, the health care professional will push the sole of your foot, bringing your toes toward you. This action is called dorsiflexion. If it produces back pain, it supports the diagnosis of nerve root pain or radiculopathy.

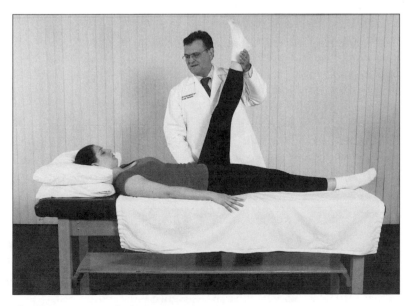

Figure 9.6   Straight leg raise test.

If pressure is present on the nerve at this foramen level, the nerve root will scream, and you will get a jolt of pain in your back. Occasionally it will produce tingling in your leg or foot. This is called a positive straight leg raise examination. It is an important part of the physical exam, telling you and your health care professional that the problem is localized at the nerve root. Therefore, it is a radiculopathy, a suffering nerve root.

Often the pain provoked during the straight leg raise is in the back of the thigh or hamstring. This is nonspecific and is not a positive straight leg raise examination. Make certain that your health care professional knows whether the pain is coming from the back or the hamstring or both. If it is a nerve root, the voice of the nerve is a jolt of pain. You will know it unequivocally. If there is some equivocation, then the problem may not be a nerve root, but this does not rule it out. Several studies show a positive straight leg exam means that significant pressure is on the nerve root in 86 percent of cases.

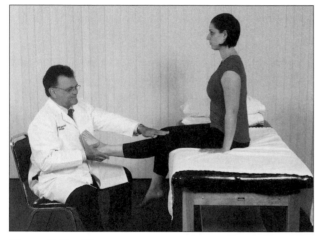

Figure 9.7   Flip test.

Flip Test

The flip test is a variation of the straight leg raise test, but it is performed while you are sitting up. The flip test is done if there is a question about the validity of the straight leg test. Sit up straight with your back arched. Lift one leg at a time (figure 9.7). If this maneuver reproduces the same pain that you feel while lying down, the test is positive.

FABER Test

The second maneuver is the FABER, or Patrick, test. FABER stands for flexion (F), abduction (AB), and external rotation (ER).

Put the heel of one foot on the knee of the other straight leg and let your bent knee drop in abduction (figure 9.8). If your motion is restricted and your knee won't abduct without causing pain in the hip area, the pain is from the hip joint. At times, this test can cause groin pain that may be from several sources, anything from a hernia to pelvic mass or lower abdominal problems.

Pain in the hip means a positive test. A positive FABER test is mainly a sign of hip degeneration or disease in the hip. If you have a positive FABER test, your health care

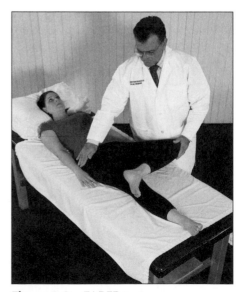

Figure 9.8   FABER test.

professional may have you lie down and externally rotate the leg outward (turn your foot out as far as it will go) to confirm the diagnosis of severe disease.

Often palpation over the hip, the greater trochanteric bursa, will provoke pain or tenderness. This result tells the health care professional that the pain is probably from a joint rather than from the back. Occasionally, more than one problem may be present.

Cervical spine maneuvers (table 9.3) are performed after ROM testing and palpation. Maneuvers include

1. range of motion (ROM),
2. Spurling maneuver,
3. Bikele maneuver (nerve root),
4. Adson's maneuver (cervical plexus injury), and
5. Tinel's sign (peripheral nerve).

Other tests may be used as well.

Table 9.3 Cervical Maneuvers

Maneuver		Sign of positive test	Specificity	Location
Spurling maneuver	Extend the neck or put pressure where the nerve root exists	Test reproduces pain, numbness, or tingling.	75 percent	Nerve root that originates in the neck
Adson's maneuver	Extend the arm to the side and raise it above the shoulder	Test causes pain or tingling down the arm.	50 percent	Nerve near the collarbone or armpit
Tinel's sign	Tap one wrist or elbow	Test causes shocklike sensation over the tapped nerve.	90 percent	Wrist or elbow
Bikele maneuver	Extend and abduct the arm with the thumb up as if hitchhiking	Test reproduces sharp pain down the arm.	50 percent	Nerve root

The pain in your neck may be caused by a nerve, joint, or muscle or may not be in the spine at all but in the thoracic outlet, the area between your neck and arm under your collarbone.

Cervical Maneuvers

Range of Motion (ROM)

Range of motion testing is important both to identify which movements cause pain and to show whether ROM is simply decreased. Your participation is important. Tell the doctor if it hurts.

Bikele Maneuver

The Bikele maneuver is like the straight leg test of the neck. The arm is stretched out straight to the side away from the body. The hand is palm up, and the thumb is stretched back like the hitchhiker's signal. A positive test causes a jolt of pain in the neck or down the arm. Its specificity is less than 50 percent, but a positive result is very helpful.

Spurling Maneuver

In the Spurling maneuver, extension in a particular direction and palpation over a particular spinous area where the nerve root exits from the cervical canal cause a shock down the arm with tingling. The test has a high specificity. Again, you must tell your doctor where and how it hurts or whether you feel numbness to help her or him reach a proper diagnosis.

Adson's Maneuver

The Adson's maneuver tells your doctor whether the problem is near your collarbone, called a thoracic outlet syndrome. The test is positive if raising your arm out and above your shoulder produces tingling in your arm and your doctor notes that your pulse disappears. This means that some structure is pressing on your nerves or blood vessel. People with long necks or people who are extremely muscular can be candidates for this syndrome. Typical symptoms include tingling and pain when the arm is raised above the head, as when brushing hair. This test is critical; many needless surgeries and medical treatments have been performed because this diagnosis was missed. An EMG can affirm this diagnosis.

Tinel's Sign

In this test the nerve that is exposed in the arm, most commonly at the elbow or at the wrist on the palm side, is tapped. A positive test occurs when tapping a particular area on the wrist or elbow causes an electric shocklike or buzzing feeling in that spot that may radiate down or up the nerve. A positive test at the elbow is highly suggestive of nerve irritability or injury of the ulnar nerve, called cubital (cube) tunnel syndrome. This irritated nerve at the elbow is most commonly caused by leaning on it or repetitive injury from talking on the telephone, especially a cell phone. The irritated nerve frequently causes tingling in the fourth and fifth fingers and is provoked when the arm is fully flexed.

A patient may be asked to mimic using a cell phone with the arm fully flexed, holding the position for one minute to see whether this activity reproduces the symptoms. This is called the Fort cell sign.

The most common tapping maneuver or Tinel's sign is at the wrist. This positive test indicates carpal tunnel syndrome, characterized by numbness especially in the thumb and index finger, frequent pain in the wrist at night, or worse pain in the morning that is made better by shaking the hand. Use of a carpal tunnel splint can help this condition.

Neurological Examination

The neurological exam is essential to identify the serious causes of low back and cervical pain. The neurological exam includes motor evaluation, sensory evaluation, reflex examination, and a gait evaluation.

Patient participation is essential for a successful neurological examination. Often the answer may include several possibilities. For example, the index finger may be numb because of a C6 root problem in the neck or carpal tunnel in the wrist. Besides simply cooperating as best you can, you also must challenge your health care professional. If part of your history includes sensory or strength loss in an extremity, pain below the knee or beyond the shoulder, or low back problems, ask your health care professional to make sure that he or she clearly understands the part of your neck or back that is involved. If he or she is unprepared to answer, ask for a second opinion.

Sensory Problems   Ask your health care professional what nerve is involved if she or he notes a sensory loss in a particular part of your body or you note one during the examination. Again, your participation is crucial. Tell your health care professional if you experience decreased or altered sensation in a particular part of your body or if it just does not feel the same. For example, if you touched a part of your body with a pin and felt an electric shock or wavelike pain spread from that area or it is hypersensitive compared with other areas, this indicates nerve impairment. Decreased sensation, altered sensation, hypersensation, or no sensation can all be signs of nerve injury. If your health care professional cannot give you a definitive answer, a specialist might help. Most health care professionals will gladly refer you for a second opinion. A good health care professional always recognizes her or his limitations. It is good medicine to transfer your case to another specialist. We are all a team—you and your health care professionals.

Motor Weaknesses   The most frequently misinterpreted symptom is weakness. Weakness can mean fatigue, a general feeling of having no get up and go. To a health care professional, weakness means decreased strength in a particular part of the body with a clear anatomical location. For example, a cervical or neck seventh root injury will cause weakness in the triceps muscle. A peroneal injury causes a dropped foot. Depression or other medical conditions can cause generalized fatigue. Diffuse weakness can be the sign of statins, which are used to combat high cholesterol.

If you think that a muscle or movement is weaker or note that a muscle group is weak during your physical exam, ask your health care professional what nerve is causing the weakness. Be sure to let your health care professional know whether the weakness is because of pain. For example, tennis elbow, an inflammation called epicondylitis, might cause you to be unable to hold a carton of milk or turn a key because of the pain of the condition. When the health care professional tests your wrist extension or grip strength, it may appear weak, but this weakness may not be because of a loss of nerve function. Your body is trying to prevent pain in the joint or over the tendon.

Know what to ask regarding your health care professional's knowledge of the localization of the neurological abnormality and be ready to let him or her know your pain is interfering with your ability to cooperate on your strength evaluation. If your health care professional cannot clearly localize and identify the spine structure, an MRI or CT scan may only confuse the diagnosis. An EMG can clarify it. Often an EMG is a sensitive test for weakness and sensory losses.

Remember that 95 percent of spinal pain resolves itself within weeks, but it recurs in 84 percent of cases, within a year in 44 percent of cases. With proper preventive care, such as the lifestyle changes discussed in chapter 5 and the body mechanics and office ergonomics advice given in chapters 6 and 7, further problems can be averted. The other 5 percent of spinal pain cases have progressive conditions that can lead to permanent disability, and 32 percent of cases may develop chronic pain. These patients need the intervention of a specialist in spine care. Their symptoms include numbness, weakness, and bowel and bladder difficulties. These patients should see a neurologist, neurosurgeon, or a spine surgeon. For those who have spinal pain but no neurological history or symptoms and who show a normal neurological exam, a chiropractor, physical therapist, exercise physiologist, a general practitioner, internist, or others can provide noninvasive and safe treatment.

If sensory, motor, or bowel and bladder symptoms do appear, don't be afraid to ask your health care professional for an evaluation by a medical specialist. If weakness or bowel and bladder problems progress, insist on being seen immediately. If you do not get satisfaction, an emergency room will call in a specialist for you.

Generally in nerve root injury, pain in the extremities is more intense than pain in the neck or back. Table 9.4 provides some general indications of the pain experienced and sensory and motor changes that occur at each spine root level.

Table 9.4 Identifying Neck and Low Back Nerve Root Symptoms

Neck nerve roots				
Nerve root	Pain in the neck and . . .	Numbness or tingling	Weakness	Other causes
Cervical 5	Front and side of the shoulder	Over shoulder	Shoulder girdle	Thoracic outlet, axillary nerve
Cervical 6	Shoulder to biceps	Thumb	Biceps	Thoracic outlet, carpal tunnel
Cervical 7	Back of the shoulder and side of the forearm	Second and third fingers	Triceps	Saturday night palsy, carpal tunnel
Cervical 8	Back of the shoulder, back of the arm, and side of the forearm	Fourth and fifth fingers	Hand	Ulnar or cubital tunnel syndrome

Low back nerve roots				
Nerve root	Pain in the back and . . .	Numbness or tingling	Weakness	Other causes
Lumbar 3 and 4	Front and side of the thigh	Front and side of the thigh	Stairs, getting up from chair	Lumbosacral plexus or femoral nerves
Lumbar 4	Shin	Shin	Turning foot inward and up	Lumbosacral plexus
Lumbar 5	Back and side of the thigh or leg	Top of foot or first toe	Drop foot, weakness in first toe	Lumbosacral plexus
Sacral 1	Back of the thigh or heel	Fifth toe	Weak calf	Piriformis syndrome

Laboratory Tests

Lab tests should prove what the doctor already suspects after her or his evaluation of your history and your physical examination. Beware of a health care professional who orders tests without giving you a good reason for the test.

Some tests are highly sensitive, and others are highly specific. High sensitivity means the test rarely misses a problem but often includes a lot of normals. One professor told me that a highly sensitive test is like a shotgun; it hits everything. A test that is specific when positive hits only the target.

A highly specific test means that if the test is positive, the likelihood is very high that you have a problem at that location. But because the test is not highly sensitive, it may miss some problems. For example, MRI and CAT scans are extremely sensitive but often not specific. In this chapter we cover noninvasive tests. Invasive tests are covered in chapter 11.

Tests can be characterized as

- laboratory tests, such as blood or urine tests;
- electrodiagnostic tests for nerve and muscle disease;
- imaging tests, including those that expose you to X-rays, such as CT scans or bone scans with radio isotopes; or
- non-X-ray tests, such as MRI scans or echograms.

Table 9.5 summarizes five common laboratory tests. *Purpose* explains the information that your doctor will learn from the test. *Specificity* refers to the accuracy of the test. *Preparation* notes what you need to do to get ready for the test. The column on exposure reveals what level of radiation you will be exposed to during the test. The column on dangers explains whether you need to be concerned about injuries that may occur because of the test. Time is the amount of time needed for the procedure, not counting any waiting time.

In this section you will learn what information each test provides to your health care professional, the underlying indications for each test, the potential dangers of the tests, and what you can do to prepare yourself for these tests.

We want to alleviate your apprehension about these tests. Your health care professional may tell you that there is nothing to the test, but she or he doesn't have to go through it. The greatest fear is not knowing what to expect.

Blood Tests

The following blood tests help the doctor know whether some general body problem, such as rheumatoid arthritis, infection, shingles, or cancer, may be present.

1. Erythrosedimentation (ESR) and C-reactive protein (CRP) tests are used to diagnose bacterial or viral infections. They are also useful to determine inflammation, such as that caused by a rheumatological disease such as ankylosing spondylitis, which causes severe spinal deformity, or lupus, a vascular inflammatory disease that causes muscle and joint pain like fibromyalgia. Missing a diagnosis such as infection or lupus can be fatal.

Table 9.5 Laboratory Tests

Test	Purpose	Specificity	Preparation	Exposure to radiation	Dangers	Time
MRI	Creates a picture of soft structures such as nerves and muscles, spinal fluid, and fat. Bone is also seen.	Only 50 percent in those over 50	None unless patient is claustrophobic and needs sedation. Patient must remain motionless for more than 20 minutes.	None. Uses magnets and radio waves. Patient must not wear any metal.	To kidneys if contrast dye is requested. Have kidney function evaluated before testing.	20 to 60 minutes
CT scan	Creates a picture of hard structures such as bone. Soft structures are not seen as well as they are with an MRI.	Only 50 percent in those over 50	None. Patient must remain motionless for 1 to 5 minutes.	Modest exposure to X-rays.	To kidneys if contrast dye is requested. Have kidney function evaluated before testing.	1 to 5 minutes
EMG	Evaluates electric response from nerves and muscles.	95 percent when done by a qualified physician	None. Patient lies on a normal exam table and can move about freely.	None.	None. Rarely causes bruising.	15 to 30 minutes
X-ray	Creates a picture of bones and their relationships to each other.	98 percent for fracture and bone alignment	None. Patient remains motionless for 5 to 20 seconds.	Yes.	X-ray exposure.	1 to 5 minutes
Bone scan	Finds areas of inflammation from arthritis, infection, or tumors.	Less than 50 percent, often nonspecific	Varies.	Yes. Note allergy to iodine.	X-ray exposure.	Varies

2. Complete blood count (CBC) is used to rule out infections or blood loss from anemia, which might indicate a colon problem, tumor, or bleeding because of an ulcer.

3. BUN, creatinine, and GFR tests are tests of kidney function. They are needed if you are going to be injected with a dye. For an MRI or CT scan, they are especially important if you take a lot of pain medications, such as Tylenol or acetaminophen.

4. Tumor markers (PSA, C-125, and CEA) are specific tests that may be ordered based on your history. Men over 40 should have a PSA done yearly. Women over 40 should have regular mammograms. Remember that 8 percent of women will get breast cancer and 12 percent of men will get prostate cancer. When these cancers spread, both go right for the spine. Unfortunately, the first sign of these cancers may be spine pain.

Electrodiganostic Tests

Electrodiagnostic tests (EDT) may provide the most specific information regarding your spine pain, especially if it involves the nerve. An electromyography (EMG) will identify the actual voice of nerve damage. The health care professional can actually hear the nerve and see its visual counterpart.

EDTs are probably the most underutilized test, but they give the most specific information about nerve involvement in spine pain. The most common electrodiagnostic tests are electromyography (EMG) and nerve conduction velocity (NCV). These are two separate exams.

Electromyography (EMG)   The EMG is a study of the nerve and muscle. This test has high specificity but low sensitivity. If the EMG is positive, there is a 98 percent chance that you have a nerve or muscle abnormality. Because the test has low sensitivity, the test will sometimes be normal even when you do have nerve irritation. A negative exam, however, may mean that the nerve involvement is not serious at present.

An EMG test is different than an imaging test such as an MRI or CT scan. An imaging test will tell your doctor what your spine looks like. An EMG test will tell him or her how your spine is functioning.

The EMG will reveal with high specificity whether a nerve is injured, accurately locate the nerve injury, and reveal the severity of the injury. After you begin treatment, an EMG can help your health care professional know the effectiveness of the treatment.

An EMG requires no specific preparation. Take your medication as usual; even anticoagulants are fine. An EMG is mildly painful, producing about the same amount of pain as acupuncture. Extremely fine needles are inserted into each muscle myotomal group (each spinal root goes to a specific muscle). An EMG takes 10 to 30 minutes per limb. No anesthesia is used, and you can drive home after the test unless your health care professional advises otherwise, which is rare.

The EMG is an essential part of your diagnosis. It will tell your doctor whether more than one condition is causing your symptoms. The incidence of poor surgical outcomes goes up by 50 percent when a neuropathy is present. If surgery is anticipated, always have an EMG performed.

Nerve Conduction Velocity (NCV)   To perform the nerve conduction velocity test, the doctor places small electrodes on certain areas to stimulate the nerve going to the area to be examined. The test causes mild to moderate discomfort at most and takes two to five minutes.

In acute spine pain, an EMG will not give accurate information for two to three weeks, because it takes that long for an injury of a nerve root to cause the muscle to show changes of that injury. Nerve conduction can be done immediately after an injury and give specific information. NCV tests are used to diagnose neuropathies, both general (diabetic) and compression neuropathy from a specific nerve injury, such as carpal tunnel (median nerve).

Magnet Resonance Image (MRI)   An MRI scan takes an image of the spine, especially showing the soft tissues of the nerves, discs, ligaments, muscles, and the spinal cord in the cervical area or cauda equina in the lumbosacral area. An MRI is less diagnostic at evaluating bone than the CT scan but can give more accurate evaluation of soft tissues. The MRI uses radio waves and powerful magnets, not X-rays. Therefore, it does not expose you to X-rays. An MRI is dangerous, however, for patients with electrical devices, such as pacemakers or defibrillators, or pumps for medications. As you can imagine, you don't want to have powerful magnets aimed at you if you have metal in you.

MRIs are indicated for acute back injury, especially if there are spinal cord or nerve compression signs at the foramen with sensory, motor, or bowel and bladder symptoms. It is an emergency if serious weakness and numbness or paralysis is occurring.

For those with chronic low back pain, an MRI scan is indicated when a tumor, infection, or other mass is suspected, or the low back pain is chronic with a history of sensory and motor complaints. For a patient who has recurrent low back pain after surgery, an MRI scan with contrast may identify scarring or infection.

Before undergoing an MRI, let your health care professional know whether you are claustrophobic or have a history of panic attacks. While in the machine, your shoulders may touch the sides and the roof may be only inches above your nose. Open MRIs are available, and the newer MRIs are less confining.

The time in the machine may vary from 20 to 60 minutes. A technician is available at all times. If necessary, you could wiggle out of the machine by yourself. Technicians are accommodating and will immediately remove you if you are uncomfortable. Often a contrast MRI scan is ordered if you have had prior surgeries or if infection is suspected. Kidney and liver function tests are advised.

If you have issues with panic attacks or are claustrophobic, you may ask whether an open scanner could be used. An open scanner sacrifices some accuracy in the image but may be sufficient for what the doctor needs. Mild tranquilizers, such as benzodiazepine, can be administered a half hour before the procedure. In rare cases, a radiologist or anesthesiologist can be available to sedate you.

An MRI scan can be noisy. Earphones with music are available. Unless you are sedated for the MRI, you can safely drive yourself home.

Computer Tomography (CT) Scan   The CT scan also provides an image of the spine. It is performed using X-ray technology and computer analysis. A CT scan is indicated for acute fractures or if bone pathology, such as a tumor, is suspected. Also, a CT scan may be indicated for a patient who is claustrophobic and does not want to be sedated.

Rarely is any preparation needed, because you are not placed in a restricted machine. Most scans take no more than one to five minutes. You are in and out before you know it.

Sometimes a health care professional will request the use of a contrast dye. Before a contrast dye is used, you should have your kidney function evaluated. If your doctor orders a CT scan with dye, ask whether you need a test of your kidney function.

X-Ray   X-rays are familiar to nearly everyone. An X-ray is indicated if degenerative or arthritic disease or fracture is suspected, when spine instability is suspected, if osteoporosis or a soft-tissue mass is suspected, or when checking for scoliosis or kyphosis. No preparation is needed. For spine instability, a flexion and extension study is performed. Flexion and extension studies are often overlooked but they are vital especially for the neck if you have rheumatoid arthritis.

Prescription

The last part of the HELP anagram stands for prescription or treatment. After analyzing the patient's history (H), the results of the physical exam (E), and the feedback from the laboratory tests (L), a prescription (P) for treatment is made. Your doctor should be able to describe how your symptoms correlate with the physical exam and the lab tests. For example, imagine a patient who has pain in the right leg, numbness in the right large toe, and a drop foot when he walks. These symptoms indicate a right L5 nerve root problem. If the EMG or MRI shows a problem to this nerve root, that diagnosis is unequivocal and the treatment can begin.

The prescription, or treatment, may be noninvasive, such as physical therapy, or invasive, such as injections or surgery. If the doctor knows that the problem is just arthritis, chiropractic treatments, physical therapy, anti-inflammatory medication, and core exercise programs are in order. If the problem is spinal canal stenosis or a damaged nerve root, invasive measures may be needed. Most important is that you receive the proper treatment for your symptoms and anatomical abnormality. Proper treatment will get you better faster and, most important, prevent further harm.

CHAPTER

10

Taking Medication for Spinal Pain

Medication is one part of spine treatment, but it is not a treatment in itself. Medication must be combined with skills such as physical therapy, chiropractic treatment, and exercise to prevent or improve back and neck pain. These skills, which were discussed in part II, are the most important means to prevent back and neck problems and treat most types of pain. Medication is best used as temporary assistance in treatment. Medication must be used only for a compelling therapeutic reason, not as a crutch.

In this chapter, we discuss

- when medication is appropriate for back and neck pain,
- what medications are best for acute pain,
- what medications are best for chronic pain,
- what the side effects are, and
- what medications may worsen symptoms or create additional problems.

Medication is the most frequent treatment by far for back and neck pain. In fact, on the first visit there is a 92 percent chance that a doctor will write a prescription for pain relief. But is that the best remedy? Blindly ordering medication is like getting rid of the smoke rather than putting out the fire. Pain is the result of a symptom. We must ask whether masking the pain will create more problems later if the injury causing the pain persists and does irreparable damage or even whether medications are the cause of chronic pain. Are the potential side effects worth the pain relief?

The medications discussed in this chapter constitute only a partial list of the medications available. The dosages, usages, and side effects described in this chapter are based on the best information available when the chapter was written, but drug usages and warning change constantly. Always consult your doctor or pharmacist to get a complete list of side effects and medication interactions.

For example, opioids such as Vicodin and Demerol can lead to both physical and psychological addiction. Anyone suffering from chronic pain and those who live with them agree that fatigue, depression, irritability, occupational limitations, and relationship struggles appear in the aftermath of excessive drug use.

In this chapter you will find a concise guide to the medications that treat back and neck problems. Pharmacological treatment should have these three objectives besides pain relief:

1. Treat the cause of the pain (for example, stopping or decreasing the inflammatory process associated with spine injury)

2. Increase pain tolerance by increasing hormones and neurotransmitters and blocking pain generators called nociceptors

3. Suppress pain that causes sleep loss and stress, which impair the immune system and pain modulating hormones, thus retarding recovery

The physician and patient must understand the benefits and the burdens of medication. The physician's job is to be knowledgeable about the process causing the pain and prescribe the proper medications to improve the problem. The doctor must also help the patient be aware of the risks and benefits of that medication and explain how to use it appropriately. Many patients admit that they have taken over-the-counter medication or a friend's or spouse's medication. A major cause of bleeding ulcers and liver and kidney damage is taking over-the-counter pain medication without a doctor's prescription.

According to the guidelines of the American Pain Society and the American College of Physicians, "The challenge in choosing medication treatment is that each class of medication is associated with a unique balance of risks and benefits." At their initial office visit, 92 percent of patients with low back pain are prescribed one medication. More than 50 percent of patients receive two or more drugs. The most common are a nonsteroidal anti-inflammatory drug (NSAID) such as aspirin, Aleve, or Motrin and a muscle relaxant or opioid (narcotic). Also, Valium (benzodiazepam), steroids, antidepressants, and antiepileptic medications are frequently prescribed.

Mary's Cautionary Tale

When Mary complained to her doctor of severe neck pain, he gave her a muscle relaxer and codeine with acetaminophen. When her pain didn't improve, her doctor prescribed 10 milligrams of Valium and Percocet as well as a laxative to ease the constipation caused by the codeine. When she couldn't sleep, Mary took an over-the-counter sleep aid. Six weeks later, Mary sought additional help, not for her pain, which was under control, but because she was having a hard time thinking, was feeling nauseated, and had lost her appetite. Her skin had a yellow cast from jaundice, a sign of serious liver damage. Mary had been overdosing on acetaminophen, which was in two of her prescription drugs as well as the over-the-counter sleep aid that she was taking. Dangerous scenarios such as this occur frequently when medication is seen as an easy fix.

Successful treatment depends on a proper diagnosis. Because back pain is generated from many body structures—bones, ligaments, nerves, and discs—each having its own voice or pain, we must determine what structure is at fault. Other substances—neurotransmitters, dopamine, and serotonin—and other parts of the nervous system such as the thalamus act as volume controls to those voices. Therefore, a doctor should not prescribe medications and you should not use over-the-counter drugs without a clear idea of the cause for your distress. Remember that medications can help you or harm you.

For most back and neck problems, *medication alone is not the best treatment.* In most cases, the best approach is to learn to avoid the causes of pain, such as poor posture or inefficient body mechanics, build up the core musculature, and engage in physical therapy and chiropractic treatment. Remember that pain is a warning. Medication for back and neck problems should never be used to hide pain. Instead, medication should treat the cause, provide relief, and allow you to participate in therapy.

First, we review the medications that act on the perception of the pain itself (table 10.1). Second, we consider those that relieve the muscle spasms that occur as the body tries to protect itself. Third, we discuss medications that influence neurotransmitters such as serotonin, dopamine, gabamine, and norepinephrine, which can diminish pain, elevate mood, and relieve depression, which itself can cause mental pain. Fourth, we consider the side effects of medications. Finally, we consider medications that work on the neurotransmission of pain and modulate or stabilize the nerve membranes and nociceptors. This effect is important in relieving the pain from nerve injury or because of subsequent scarring after nerve root injury (pinching a nerve).

NSAIDS

NSAIDS such as Aleve, Naproxen, Motrin, and Celebrex work in the cyclooxygenase reduction-inhibiting prostaglandins that cause inflammation and sensitize peripheral nociceptors (pain-producing cells or sites). The primary reaction of NSAIDs is in decreasing nociceptor or pain-generating cell sensitivity. Studies show that if NSAIDs are used early, less alternative pain medication is needed. Use of more than one NSAID is not advised because of their potential to cause gastric upset such as heartburn. NSAIDS such as ibuprofen inhibit the action of aspirin to prevent heart attacks and stroke when taken within 14 hours of each other. If you take aspirin for heart-related reasons, remember that NSAIDs inactivate the effect of aspirin and increase the risk of heart attack and stroke.

How each medication should be taken depends on the medication's half-life. Generally, by doubling the half-life you can determine how long the drug remains in the body. Always take medication as prescribed by your doctor but be aware of its half-life.

Aspirin is metabolized in the liver, and its half-life is approximately three hours. It is excreted by the kidneys. Its main side effects are stomach upset and bleeding. Other effects are that it prevents heart attack and stroke.

Table 10.1 Medications That Act on the Perception of Pain

Name	Generic	Dose	Half-life	Pain relief rating*	Best use	Side effects	Other properties
Bayer Aspirin Anacin	Aspirin (NSAID) Salicytates	325 mg to 650 mg	3 hours	1 to 2	Acute mild to moderate pain	Stomach upset, bleeding, ulcers.	Prevents heart attack and stroke
Tylenol	Acetaminophen	500 mg	2 to 4 hours	2	Mild muscular skeletal pain, mild chronic pain, acute back pain	Chronic use can lead to kidney or liver damage. Chronic use is the number-one cause of kidney failure.	Does not ease inflammation, help with sleep, or treat the cause of pain
Advil Motrin Unpin	Ibuprofen (NSAID)	200 mg	2 hours	2.5	Joint and muscle pain, acute back pain; less effect after 7 days	Stomach ulcers.	Increases risk of heart attack and stroke
Aleve Naproxen	Naproxen (NSAID)	220 mg	12 to 24 hours	3	Acute joint and muscle pain, acute back pain; less effect after 7 days	Hypertension, stomach ulcers.	May increase risk of heart attack and stroke
Celebrex	Celecoxib (NSAID)	100 mg to 200 mg	11 hours	3.5	Acute and chronic back pain	Stomach upset is less frequent.	Increases risk of heart attack and stroke
Ultra	Tramadol	50 mg	5 1/2 to 7 hours	3.7	Acute and chronic moderate to severe back pain	Constipation, headache, drowsiness.	Seizures, respiratory problems, and depression
Vicodin Lorcet	Hydrocodone (H) and acetaminophen (A)	5 mg (H) and 500 mg (A)	4 hours (H) and 1 1/2 to 3 hours (A)	4	Moderate to severe back pain**	Constipation, drowsiness, addiction, kidney damage.	Addiction and depression
Codeine	Codeine	15, 30, or 60 mg	2 1/2 to 4 hours	4	Moderate to severe pain**	Constipation, liver damage.	Drowsiness, addiction, depression
Fentanyl	Eentanyl	50 mg to 100 mg	3 to 7 hours intramuscular, 7 hours transdermal	4 to 8	Severe pain**	Constipation, liver damage, nausea, vomiting.	Drowsiness, addiction, depression, slow heart rate

Name	Generic	Dose	Half-life	Pain relief rating*	Best use	Side effects	Other properties
Vicodin ES Lorcet Plus	Hydrocodone (H) and acetaminophen (A)	7.5 mg (H) and 650 mg (A)	4 hours (H) and 1 1/2 to 3 hours (A)	4.5	Moderate to severe back pain**	Constipation, drowsiness, addiction, kidney damage.	Addiction and depression
Demerol	Meperidine	50 mg to 100 mg	3 to 5 hours	4 to 6	Severe acute back pain**	Drowsiness, confusion.	Rapid addiction, euphoria
Lortab	Hydrocodone (H) and acetaminophen (A)	10 mg (H) and 500 mg (A)	4 hours (H) and 1 1/2 to 3 hours (A)	5	Moderate to severe back pain**	Constipation, drowsiness, addiction, kidney damage.	Addiction and depression
Norco with paracetamol	Hydrocodone (H) and acetaminophen (A)	10 mg (H) and 325 mg (A)	4 hours (H) and 1 1/2 to 3 hours (A)	5	Moderate to severe back pain**	Constipation, drowsiness, addiction, kidney damage.	Addiction and depression
Percocet	Oxycodone HCL (O) and acetaminophen (A)	10 mg (O) and 325 mg (A)	3 to 4 1/2 hours (O) and 1 1/2 to 3 hours (A)	5 to 7	Moderate to severe back pain**	Constipation, drowsiness, addiction, kidney damage.	Addiction and depression
Percodan	Oxycodone HCL (O) and aspirin (AS)	4.5 mg (O) and 325 mg (AS)	3 to 4 1/2 hours	5 to 7	Moderate to severe back pain**	Constipation, drowsiness, addiction, kidney damage.	Addiction and depression
Dilaudid	Hydromorphone	2 mg	2 to 3 hours	8	Moderate to severe back pain**	Constipation, drowsiness, addiction, kidney damage.	Addiction, depression, euphoria; may react adversely with other drugs
Oxycontin	Oxycodone HCL	10, 15, 20, 30, 40, 60, 80, or 160 mg	3 to 4 1/2 hours	8.5	Moderate to severe back pain**	Constipation, drowsiness, addiction, kidney damage.	Addiction, depression, euphoria
MS Contin	Morphine sulfate	10 to 30 mg	2 to 3 hours	10	Moderate to severe back pain**	Constipation, drowsiness, addiction, kidney damage.	Addiction, depression, euphoria

*Pain relief is factored on a scale from 1 to 10, with 1 being the least and 10 being the most. Ratings are estimates based on our review of the medical literature and personal experience.

**Use only during acute phase for no more than six weeks unless advised by your doctor. Chronic use may lead to chronic pain syndrome.

Acetaminophen has an antifever and analgesic action. It works on an area in the brain near the heat regulatory center. Acetaminophen is metabolized in the liver and has a half-life of three to four hours. It is excreted by the kidney. Its major side effects are liver and kidney damage. Because it is often combined with other analgesics, many patients are unaware that when they take acetaminophen in combination with other analgesics, such as Vicodin and Percocet, they are taking double doses of acetaminophen. Over several months, they may damage their kidneys and liver. Always check whether the medication that you are given has acetaminophen and another analgesic. Also, because most drugs are metabolized in the liver and excreted by the kidneys, liver and kidney function should be checked regularly by your doctor.

> **!** Check your prescribed medication and note if it has acetaminophen plus another analgesic. Be careful not to take double doses of acetaminophen. If you have questions, ask your doctor or pharmacist. Acetaminophen is the chief cause of liver failure in the U.S.

OPIOIDS

Morphine and other opioids bind to various opioid receptors, producing pain relief and sedation that cause loss of attention, concentration, and memory. Opioids also have been found to interfere with the normal pain threshold that is modulated by neurotransmitters, such as serotonin. Over a two-week period, an opioid can decrease your natural pain threshold, causing an increase in pain sensitivity after the opioid is discontinued. Through several mechanisms, opioids cause tolerance and a need for increasingly larger doses. Opioids also interfere with the frontal lobe, the home of executive functioning, causing the person on the medication to become ineffectual and unmotivated. Opioid use frequently leads to depression and problems at home and work. For these reasons, opioids should be used only for short periods to treat serious pain and under the strict guidance of a doctor. Opioids are metabolized in the liver and are excreted most often in the urine, bile, and feces.

Morphine and other opioids are addictive when taken chronically. The five predictors of addiction are

1. anticipatory dosing (taking medication to avoid pain even when pain is not felt),
2. decreased interest such as loss of libido or decreased socialization and physical activity,
3. slurred or monotone speech,
4. poor recall, and
5. poor hygiene and dress.

If your physician prescribes opioids for the long term—more than two months—please sit down with your doctor and discuss alternative methods of treatment or ask for a second opinion. Long-term treatment with opioids should be done only under scrutiny by a physician because addiction to opioids is a major complication and a cause of chronic back pain.

MUSCLE RELAXANTS

Muscle relaxants (table 10.2) are used to treat acute spine pain, improve range of motion, and increase blood supply to the muscles. Muscle relaxants also interrupt the pain–spasm–pain cycle. They are helpful in increasing range of motion and mobility. Muscle relaxants act either on nerve cells in the spinal cord or on the muscle spindle or cells. Some, such as Zanaflex, also inhibit prostaglandins and have an anti-inflammatory effect. They are metabolized mainly in the liver and kidneys. Often, muscle relaxants are associated with drowsiness. Those of the benzodiazepam family, such as Valium, have serious addictive qualities.

Table 10.2 Muscle Relaxants

Name	Generic	Dose	Best use	Side effects	Other properties
Soma	Carisoprodol	10 mg daily	Acute spine pain or recurrence	Drowsiness (20 percent)	Increased relief when combined with NSAIDs
Baclofen	Baclofen	10 to 80 mg daily	Chronic spasticity	Severe drowsiness (49 percent)	Best for spinal cord injury
Valium	Diazepam	10 mg	Not advised	Addictive, drowsiness	Can benefit patients who have severe panic and anxiety associated with low back pain
Zanaflex	Tizanidine	4 mg daily, increase to 3 times daily	Acute pain syndrome	Drowsiness	Inhibits both leukotriene and prostiglandins, which produce pain; few side effects if used less than 1 week
Decadron Prednisone Medrol	Corticosteroids	Varies according to type	Acute with neurological and nerve root pain	Diabetes, sleeplessness, anxiety	Be cautious of long-term use; best for joint and muscle injury; short term use is 1-2 weeks

Note: This is only a partial list of medications, dosages, side effects, and other information. Always ask your doctor and pharmacist for a complete list of side effects and medication interactions.

ANTIDEPRESSANTS

The primary mechanism of antidepressants (table 10.3) is not their antidepressant effect but the way that they filter the effect of pain perception. The brain has its own mechanism of filtering messages sent to the cortex, the awareness part of the brain. Just as you adjust a nozzle on a garden hose to change the flow of water, you can tighten or loosen the flow of pain to the brain. Fewer pain messages get to the cortex. Antidepressants are metabolized in the liver and excreted in the urine and feces. They increase norepinephrine and serotonin, thereby increasing pain threshold. At first, many patients experience side effects such as dry mouth and mild sedation. Improvement in mood follows. Other side effects are weight gain and interference with sexual performance.

Table 10.3 Antidepressants

Name	Generic	Dose	Best use	Side effects
Tricyclics				
Elavil	Amitriptyline	25 mg to 150 mg	Increase sleep and decrease depression	Dry mouth, drowsiness, urinary retention, heart arrhythmia
Sinequan	Doxepin HCL	10 mg to 100 mg	Increase sleep	Dry mouth, drowsiness, urinary retention
SSRIs				
Effexor	Venlafaxine	37.5 mg to 300 mg	Chronic low back pain	Dry mouth, drowsiness, urinary retention, sleeplessness; no cardiac side effects
Cymbalta	Duloxetine	20, 30, or 60 mg	Chronic low back pain	Seizure (rare), glaucoma, nausea, dry mouth, constipation, insomnia, sexual problems
Savella	Milnacipran	12.5 mg to 100 mg	Chronic low back pain	Seizure (rare), nausea, constipation, insomnia, sweating, weight loss, decrease in libido

Note: This is only a partial list of medications, dosages, side effects, and other information. Always ask your doctor and pharmacist for a complete list of side effects and medication interactions.

NERVE-MODULATING PAIN RELIEVERS

Nerve-modulating pain relievers (table 10.4) work by stabilizing the injured nerve membranes and decreasing the pain perception from nociceptors in various tissues. Side effects include diarrhea, drowsiness, weight loss, and, occasionally, tingling sensations and swelling of the ankles.

CORTICOSTEROIDS

Drugs such as prednisone, Medrol, and Decadron are considered the ultimate anti-inflammatories. They decrease swelling and cause a dramatic decrease in pain when the nerve is being compressed, such as with a herniated disc. Corticosteriods can decrease the pressure caused by swelling on nerves and other tissues, relieving the damaging effect on the delicate nerves in the back. In addition, corticosteriods are great inhibitors of cytokinins and prostaglandins, which cause damage to surrounding tissues.

Table 10.4 Nerve-Modulating Pain Relievers

Brand name	Generic	Dose	Best use	Side effects
Neurontin	Gabapentin	100 mg to 5,000 mg (divided doses)	Chronic back pain	Diarrhea, drowsiness
Lyrica	Pregabalin	25 mg to 300 mg (divided doses)	Chronic back pain	Tingling, burning, shocklike sensations; can cause dizziness, weight gain, swelling of limbs (increased with use of narcotics and alcohol)
Topomax	Topiromax	25 mg to 200 mg (divided doses)	Chronic back pain	Drowsiness, severe weight loss, tingling, depression

Note: This is only a partial list of medications, dosages, side effects, and other information. Always ask your doctor and pharmacist for a complete list of side effects and medication interactions.

Because long-term use can lead to serious side effects to bones, joints, and blood vessels, including hypertension and diabetes, corticosteriods should be used for short-term (one- or two-week) treatment of back and neck pain. The first indication for their use is a certain diagnosis of spinal cord or nerve injury. Often used short term (six days) in acute nerve root (radiculopathy) compression. It can be diagnostic. If it relieves the pain and symptoms, it supports the diagnosis of nerve pain.

USE PILLS WITH SKILL

For most spinal disorders, medication alone is not the best treatment. In most cases, learning specific skills is the best treatment. Learn to avoid precipitating causes such as poor posture or inadequate body mechanics. Strengthen your core through a good exercise program. Perhaps try physical therapy or chiropractic treatment.

Pain is a warning. The medication that you take for your back and neck problems should never hide the problem but should treat the cause and give you relief.

IV

Exploring Surgical Options

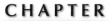

CHAPTER

Getting Injections for Spinal Pain

No one likes needles, but they can be a back pain sufferer's best friend if used by the right person for the right reason. When administered correctly, injections are as safe as crossing the street. In this chapter we discuss epidural steroid and facette joint injections given by physicians who have had additional training in providing these procedures. The discussion does not pertain to office-based, routinely performed local injections given into trigger points, bursae, or muscle.

The epidural injection delivers a steroid—a strong anti-inflammatory agent—to the epidural space. This epidural space is the layer closest to the nerve roots. Facette joint injections also deliver steroids, but they target the inflamed joint capsules or sensory nerves that supply the facette joint. These types of injections are more involved than office-based injections. They are often performed in a hospital or surgery center and require the use of an X-ray machine to help guide the needles. Often light sedation is used to make the patient comfortable during the injection procedure. In experienced hands, these injections are safe and have a low risk of complications.

INJECTION SPECIALISTS

Pain management physicians and spine surgeons perform most epidural and facet injections. Pain management physicians have extended training in prescribing narcotic and non-narcotic medicines, besides their training in the administration of injections. They have a good understanding of the benefits of physical therapy and can be of any medical subspecialty, although most tend to be spinal orthopedists, anesthesiologists, or radiologists.

Usually spine surgeons or anesthesiologists perform these injections on their own patients to help identify the location of the pain. Most often the goal is to identify which nerve root or facette joint is causing the problem. If the surgeon can identify the pain source, ultimately it can be addressed successfully with or without surgery.

DIAGNOSTIC AND THERAPEUTIC ROLES

Injections provide two main benefits. First, they provide the doctor answers about the cause of your discomfort. Second, they provide relief from pain. If the injection helps your doctor determine what is troubling you, it's called a test. When the injection gives you relief of your symptoms, it's called a procedure. Injections can serve both diagnostic and therapeutic roles. Often one injection does both.

To highlight this concept, consider the following case. Sue, a 50-year-old office assistant with two children, had pain that radiated to the front of her shin. She reported that she kept tripping because her foot was weak. A medical workup led to a diagnosis of an L4 or L5 disc level pathology, which was supported by an MRI. It was not clear which nerve root—L4 or L5—was involved. Complicating matters was the electro diagnostic test result. This test indicated a possible problem of the peroneal nerve at the knee, which may have been mimicking other symptoms often associated with the low back pathology that she was being examined for.

This case shows the value of a spinal injection. If the L4 nerve root was the source of the pain and a selective L4 nerve root block relieved all of Sue's pain, then the nerve root block had diagnostic value. It helped complete the diagnosis that the L4 nerve was the problem. Because it relieved Sue's symptoms, the injection was therapeutic as well. If the L4 nerve root block had no diagnostic value and offered no symptom relief, the injection still had merit because it saved Sue from a potentially unnecessary surgery on the L4 nerve root. Making an accurate diagnosis is the key to good medicine. These injections are a new technique that make a difference.

TYPES OF INJECTIONS

Different combinations of medicines may be injected. The most common injections are a numbing medicine such as lidocaine or marcaine and a steroid such as Depo-Medrol. The numbing medicine has an immediate effect, making the procedure less painful by numbing the tissues being poked with the needle. The steroid is a strong anti-inflammatory agent that decreases inflammation around the structure being injected.

There are many types of injections. Many people are familiar with the term *epidural*. Most injections for the back are epidural in nature, but others are not. They are broken down by region of the spine: cervical (neck), thoracic (chest), and lumbar (low back). They are categorized by the direction of the needle's approach: interlaminar, transforaminal (figure 11.1), or caudal (figure 11.2). They can go into the facette joint (figure 11.3) or can block the nerve to the facette joint. Facette nerve blocks can be especially helpful. If they are successful in reducing a patient's pain, that nerve can be killed in a procedure called a rhizotomy. You need not fear this result; your body will get along just fine without the irritated and symptom-producing nerve. In fact, you'll often feel much better.

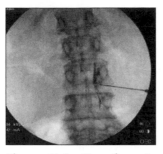

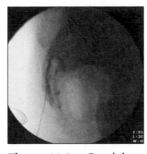

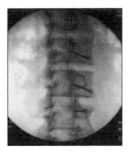

Figure 11.1 Transforaminal epidural injection. The black line is the needle entering the transforaminal space.

Figure 11.2 Caudal epidural injection. The black line is the needle entering the sacral hiatus near the tailbone.

Figure 11.3 Unilateral facette joint injections. The black lines are the tips of the needles at the base of each facette joint.

PREPARATION

After your physician decides that an injection is appropriate, follow these guidelines to make the experience easier. Some physicians provide light sedation, called twilight anesthesia, whereas others administer injections using local anesthesia only. If you will be given a twilight sedation, you must not eat or drink anything after midnight the night before the injection. Additionally, you'll be slightly groggy afterward so you'll need to arrange for a driver to transport you to and from the center where the injection will be performed.

If you are taking blood thinners such as Coumadin, Heparin, Lovenox, or Plavix, your physician will have you discontinue them 5 to 10 days before the procedure. If your blood is too thin, it won't clot properly, which can lead to excessive bleeding in and around the zone where the injection is performed.

INJECTION DAY

On the morning of the injection, take your normal medications, except for blood thinners, using the smallest volume of water possible. Be sure to take your blood pressure medications so that you are not hypertensive when you show up at the facility. Also, verify your transportation arrangements because you may still be groggy after the injection.

When you arrive at the facility, you will need to register. Personal demographic and insurance information will be requested and reviewed. Depending on the patient volume and the efficiency of the facility, this process may take 20 to 60 minutes. After you check in, nurses will review your medical history and have you change into a hospital gown. They will perform a cursory exam, begin an intravenous (IV) line to administer fluids, and collect any blood or urine samples as needed. Because injections often are performed with the assistance of X-ray radiation, women of reproductive age usually are screened for pregnancy before the injection.

When your turn comes, you'll be taken into the procedure room. Usually injections are performed as you lie face down, but they can be done while you are seated or lying on your side as well. After you are in position, the administration of the IV medication will begin and the injection will start. Some injections are performed with the patient completely sedated, whereas others require some level of patient response. In these situations, less sedating medicine is given through the IV so that you can verbalize your feedback regarding leg, arm, neck, or back pain. The actual injection procedure will take a few minutes to half an hour.

After the injection is done, you will be taken to a recovery room to revive from the anesthesia. Nurses will monitor your heart rate, blood pressure, and respiration rate. After your vital signs are stable, you'll be cleared for discharge to go home.

POSTINJECTION RECOVERY

The most common side effect is some muscle soreness in the area where the injection was performed. Often ice and anti-inflammatory medications such as Aleve or Advil help with this soreness and pain. Typically, the muscle soreness, if present, goes away in a few days.

A risk of infection or bleeding occurs anytime the skin is broken, as happens when a needle is used. These risks are low with injections. Common signs of an infection are redness, warmth, tenderness, pus drainage from the injection site, or a fever of 101 degrees Fahrenheit (38.3 degrees Celsius) or greater. If you have any of these symptoms, contact your physician immediately. The risk of bleeding is extremely low. The size of the needle for the injection is about the size of an average sewing needle and causes minimal damage. With proper blood clotting, there is little to worry about. If you experience persistent bleeding, direct pressure over the site often will stop the bleeding. When in doubt, contact your physician.

Another potential complication is a spinal headache. The nerve tissue that runs up and down the bony spinal canal is bathed by cerebrospinal fluid. The nerves and the spinal fluid are contained in a long, flexible tubular sac that also spans the length of the spinal canal. If the sac is punctured, spinal fluid may leak out. The lowered volume of cerebrospinal fluid may produce a headache that worsens when you stand erect as more fluid leaks out of the hole. The headache may go away if you lie completely flat or horizontal. Lying flat reduces the pressure and limits the amount of fluid that leaks from the injection hole. Lying down for 24 hours cures the problem in 90 percent of cases. If the headaches remain, another intervention called a blood patch may be needed.

Occasionally, you may feel some numbness or tingling in the legs. This condition is related to the numbing medication component, often lidocaine or marcaine, of the injection. Rarely, you may feel weak in the legs, similar to a mild paralysis. When you first stand up after the injection, be sure to proceed slowly and stand within arm's reach of a chair or stretcher. In the event that your legs are not strong enough to support your weight, you may need an object nearby for assistance. Numbness and weakness symptoms are common and are related to how sensitive you are to the numbing medication. They will resolve within several minutes to several hours. Don't worry; before discharge from the hospital you will be walking again.

Serious complications to epidural injections are rare but can occur. Side effects requiring immediate care include neurological changes, bleeding, and infection. Contact your physician if you experience any of the side effects discussed. Table 11.1 reviews the more common and relevant side effects and provides detail about what to do. When in doubt, contact your doctor. She or he can't help you if you don't reveal what you're experiencing.

Immediately after the epidural injection, patients often note some immediate relief that lasts only a few hours. This short-term effect is expected and is related to the numbing medicine component of the concoction. Anywhere from two to seven days later, depending on how your body reacts, the anti-inflammatory component of the injection concoction will begin to take effect. As the steroid decreases the inflammation and irritation around the nerves, the pain will begin to subside. This delayed effect is important to note and report to your physician at your follow-up. The American Academy of Neurology states lumbosacral epidurals will provide pain relief for one to six weeks.

Table 11.1   Common Side Effects to Injections to Treat Back and Neck Pain

Side effect	Remedy	When to call the doctor
Positional headache (for example, a headache that worsens when you stand but eases when you lie down)	Lie flat in bed and rest; possibly have a blood patch applied	Immediately; headache may be related to dural puncture and may a require blood patch.
Fever greater than 10 °F (38.3 °C)	Take Tylenol	Immediately; fever may be a sign of infection.
Bowel or bladder dysfunction (for example, the inability to void urine or stool)	May require tests such as an MRI to further identify the dysfunction	Immediately; bowel or bladder dysfunction may be a sign of compression on the nerves.
Weakness in extremities	May require tests such as an MRI to further identify the weakness	Immediately; weakness may be a sign of compression on the nerves.
Bleeding	Apply pressure to the area	Immediately; bleeding usually slows unless the patient has an underlying bleeding disorder or is on a blood thinner such as Coumadin.
Numbness, tingling, and pain in extremities	Observation initially	Within 72 hours; not urgent.
Pain at the injection site	Tylenol, NSAIDs, ice, observation initially	Within 72 hours; not urgent.
Nonpositional headaches	Tylenol, NSAIDs	Within 72 hours; not urgent.

FOLLOW UP

After the injection, your doctor will want to know whether it was helpful. Simply tell him or her what you feel. Only you know. If the injection did not help at all, report that. This information will provide clues for your doctor to look for other sources of the pain. On the other hand, if the injection helped, whether partially or completely, temporarily or permanently, then report that. This information lets your doctor know that the injection site is a potential source of the pain, which will help guide treatment. Whatever the result, let your doctor know exactly how you feel. Giving answers that you think your doctor wants to hear will be misleading if they are not accurate. Simply tell him or her how you feel, and you'll be that much closer to reducing your spinal discomfort.

Although patients and physicians alike hope that the effects of the injection will last forever, often they do not. In fact, relief may last from several hours to several years, most commonly from two to six weeks. The duration of the response depends on several variables, the most important of which are the extent of the disease, your response to the steroid, and your progress with physical therapy after the injections. Many studies document the benefits of epidural or facette joint injections. A reasonable success expectation is that more than 70 percent of patients will receive greater than 50 percent pain relief after a series of three injections.

To get a full effect, a series of three injections is often performed. If after the third injection only marginal improvement has been experienced, a fourth or fifth injection is unlikely to be beneficial. At this point, you and your doctor will need to decide whether surgery is appropriate. (See chapter 12 for more on surgical intervention.)

Classic medical teaching dictates that you can receive three epidural injections per year per condition, but a physician may recommend fewer or more based on the individual patient's medical status, symptoms, and severity of structural abnormality. For example, if a patient has a large disc herniation that is causing severe pain and weakness, the physician may recommend a simple surgery to remove the herniation rather than subject the patient to a protracted course of epidurals staged every 2 weeks only to have the surgery 6 to 12 weeks later. Conversely, if an elderly, medically fragile patient is too sick to undergo surgery, continuance of epidural injections beyond three per year would be appropriate if there is an ongoing benefit. These are just a couple of scenarios in which the physician might deviate from the three-per-year rule.

Injecting more than three times a year becomes problematic because of complications arising from the quantity of steroid given over the course of the treatments. Predicting the dosage of steroid that will lead to medical complications in any one person is difficult, so the three-per-year rule is generally adhered to.

Epidural injections are a safe and effective way for your physician to locate symptom-producing structures while providing you relief. When done properly, injections have minimal complications. When you follow up with your doctor, be sure to tell her or him exactly how you feel. Even telling your physician that you have experienced no relief has merit because that result tells your physician to look elsewhere for the cause of your pain. Epidurals and facette joint injections provide diagnostic value in addition to symptom relief. Sometimes, in spite of all the right therapies, ergonomics, and self-administered first aid, the body needs a little outside intervention to help it heal. We hope that this information on injections will ease your mind about the process if an injection is recommended for you.

CHAPTER

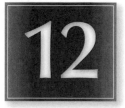

12

Considering Surgery

Most patients, whether they are Olympic or professional athletes, weekend warriors, business persons, secretaries, grandfathers, or grandmothers, have two questions: What is wrong, and can it be fixed? The second question, whether it can be fixed, causes the most anxiety, because surgery may be needed. Surgery is usually the last thing patients want, and it should be a last resort, performed only under careful consultation and scrutiny. The consultation with a spinal surgeon depends on the HELP model (see chapter 9, page 143), a thorough review of your history, a physical examination, laboratory tests, and prescription. The prescription is the advised treatment, whether medical or surgical.

In this chapter, we explore the compelling, strong, and relative indications for surgery. If surgery is needed, you will learn how to discuss this option with your surgeon and the risks, complications, and benefits that you can expect. We cover the alternatives to surgery that might be tried first and the best techniques and approaches to use for your specific problem. Remember that one surgical procedure does not fit all. We also discuss trust and ways to evaluate your spinal surgeon. Does your surgeon have a team that helps with follow-up during or after surgery, a team of the best specialists ready on the spot to help you? Will your surgeon be there for you whatever the outcome? The surgery itself is crucial, of course, but the entire procedure is important, including pre-op and post-op care. Surgery is not to be taken lightly, but it should not be avoided when it is necessary.

Let's discuss the most important question first. When is surgery indicated, and what criteria does the surgeon use?

CONSIDERATIONS FOR SURGERY

Indications for surgery are classified as compelling, strong, or relative reasons. Compelling indications mean that if surgery is not done, you will be left with a permanent loss of function, pain, or both. Strong indications mean that if surgery is not done, you may suffer a significant loss of function or continued severe pain. Relative indications mean that surgery may be done because of life necessities or to enhance quality of life when alternatives such as physical therapy and spinal injections have failed. This justification may apply to professional athletes, working mothers, construction workers, or those whose quality of life inspires them to choose surgery.

Surgery as an exploratory option is not a relative indication. Always seek a second opinion if this is what your surgeon advises.

Compelling Indications

Compelling indications may occur suddenly or come on gradually. They include weakness that corresponds to an identifiable location in the spine, such as a herniated disc or spinal stenosis. A herniated disc is an expulsion of the insides of the multilayered elastic fibrous tissue (the annulus fibrosa) into the spinal canal where the nerves lie. Spinal stenosis is a narrowing of the spinal canal where the spinal cord or the cauda equina (end of the spinal cord) exits. You may have loss of bladder or bowel function or control, the onset of which corresponds to the spine problem. You may experience sensory symptoms that are persistent and feel like pins and needles or burning, or you may have a loss of sensation associated with the weakness and bowel or bladder loss. Pain is often sharp, piercing, and electric, radiating down the arm or leg. Arm or leg pain is often more intense than neck or back pain. A final compelling indication is an unstable spine segment that moves when you bend forward (flexion) or backward (extension). An unstable spine causes the bone and ligaments to injure the nerves when the body moves.

Alice's story demonstrates compelling indications for surgery. Alice is a 42-year-old executive secretary. She went to her doctor after eight weeks of arm pain that was more intense than her neck pain. The pain was piercing down the backs of her arms and was associated with a tingling sensation to the third, fourth, and fifth fingers on both sides. Looking up at the ceiling provoked the pain and numbness. Also, looking up at a monitor in front of her with her arms raised occasionally provoked the same type of aching pain and numbness down the arms. Her private medical doctor prescribed a muscle relaxant and physical therapy, but this provided no relief. In the past month, her legs felt heavy and her arms were fatigued, making it difficult to type. She was referred for a surgery consultation when she realized that her hands were becoming clumsy to the point that she could no longer type. Additionally, she noted difficulty urinating two weeks earlier, especially the inability to start the flow of urine, and she was losing her balance and could not walk a straight line.

When the surgeon examined her, Alice's reflexes were extremely brisk. Looking up at the ceiling caused pain and tingling in both arms. She also noted that water in the shower was not as hot below her neck as above her neck. An MRI scan of the neck area showed that a large mass was compressing her spinal cord, a condition known as central canal stenosis, or narrowing of the canal where the spinal cord passes through the spinal canal. Alice was given the diagnosis and told the risks and benefits of surgery. The risks were compelling; she would become paralyzed unless pressure on the spinal cord was relieved. Four weeks after surgery, Alice had fully recovered and was back at work.

Unfortunately, some people wait too long. Weakness, heaviness in the arms or legs after activity, and tingling, radiating, throbbing, or piercing pain down the arms or legs, especially if the arm or leg pain is more intense than the neck or back pain, are compelling indications for surgery. When bowel or bladder problems occur, the time to wait has ended. Ask your doctor to refer you to a spine surgeon immediately. You need an immediate evaluation, not one in three or four weeks or months. Ask your doctor to call for a referral to tell them of the urgency. If any sudden progression of weakness occurs, go to the emergency room. The doctor there can call for an emergency evaluation.

Strong Indications

Strong indications include arm or leg pain on one side. You may have tried medication and other therapies, but your symptoms have progressed or returned. You are experiencing pain sufficient to prevent you from doing your job or performing normal daily activities.

Consider Fred's case. Fred is 66 years old. For the last 2 years, he has had a dull low backache. Six months ago, the pain started radiating down the backs and fronts of both legs. The pain was clearly provoked after Fred stood for 5 minutes or more or walked. Sitting provided relief. After walking a block, Fred's legs and especially his feet tingled. He noticed increasing difficulty with urination, although he thought that the problem might be because of his prostate. Fred had limited range of movement backward, and this movement worsened his pain and symptoms. An MRI showed a severe narrowing of the lumbar L4 and L5 vertebrae canal. Fred was suffering from lumbosacral spinal narrowing (stenosis), a condition that is occurring in increasing frequency in up to 6 percent of those over 60 years of age. He could not work with his wife or physically stand and talk to his business associates. He also could not find a comfortable position in which to sleep. Eight months of conservative treatment did not help, so Fred agreed to the recommended surgery. Two months later, he said, "If I had only known how great surgery would make me feel, I would have had it earlier." Fred had both compelling and strong indications for surgery, and the surgical intervention was eventually successful.

Fred was fortunate. His back pain early on would have been a strong indication for surgery, but the onset of bladder problems and the inability to walk changed his need for surgery to compelling. Not all cases progress as Fred's did. Even when progression does not occur, some patients choose surgery because of quality-of-life issues.

Sometimes patients wait too long, and nerves become damaged to the extent that surgery cannot return full function. An EMG or electrical test can reveal how badly the nerve is damaged and may predict your prognosis. Also, waiting too long may cause damage to the insulation of the nerve, causing long-term pain even after surgical intervention.

Good communication with your spinal surgeon or neurologist is essential in helping you make the correct decision. There is a time to act and a time to wait. Your spine surgeon and neuro-orthopedist can help you with that decision.

Sam's case includes strong indications for surgery. Sam is a 45-year-old executive. He developed sudden low back and leg pain after he picked up a heavy box. The leg pain was worse than the back pain. He described the pain first as the worst pain that he ever felt in his back and down his leg. Now it was a deep ache in the side of his calf. The pain was made worse by bending, lifting, or twisting. He felt numbness and weakness on his heel and the ball of his foot. He couldn't lift his left foot off the ground. After a trial of steroids and eight weeks of physical therapy, Sam's symptoms remained. Rest made it tolerable, but he could barely get through a workday. An MRI showed a large herniated disc at L5 and S1. An EMG showed injury to that nerve. In Sam's case, the history, exam, and test all agreed. Removal of the herniated disc gave Sam full relief.

In cases of strong indications such as Fred's and Sam's, medication is often prescribed to reduce nerve swelling. For example, a six-day course of prednisone or Medrol or epidural injections might be tried first unless rapid progression, strength loss, or excruciating pain occurs. Medication often relieves symptoms, but they frequently return. If these measures do not improve symptoms after a course of physical therapy or if symptoms recur, surgery should be advised to avoid permanent nerve damage and disability.

Relative Indications

Relative indications include pain without neurological deficits, such as weakness or tingling, but with an identifiable cause such as an unstable spinal segment, stenosis, disc herniation, or spondylolisthesis. You may have had prior surgeries, and the revision of the prior surgery would likely reduce pain or symptoms. You think that surgery is needed so that you can return to a higher level of activity required by your job and lifestyle.

Nick is a 35-year-old professional golfer. For 2 years, he had intermittent back pain down his leg and numbness or weakness, often provoked by his golf swing. With the help of a core exercise program, he'd been able to play with only temporary setbacks, but the pain was becoming more severe and was seriously interfering with his career. An X-ray and MRI scan showed old stress fractures of the spine and a slippage of one vertebra on the other, though it was minimal. An EMG did not show any nerve damage. After careful consideration of the risks and benefits of surgery and the potential consequences to his career, Nick elected to have surgery. Had he not golfed professionally, he probably would have not have needed surgery, but he elected to undergo a surgical procedure that could return him to competition pain free. This case demonstrates a relative need for surgery.

Other examples are a carpenter or police officer whose job requires a high level of mobility. At times, the decision may hinge on relieving chronic disabling pain. In these relative cases you need to know all you can about realistic benefits versus the risks of surgery. Surgeons are not miracle workers. To make a decision, you need communication and trust.

Myth

THERAPY DIDN'T WORK, SO I GUESS I NEED SURGERY

This statement may be true or false. Surgery is a viable option for a select number of people with a select number of conditions. In the process of making this decision, ask yourself whether your therapy so far has been good therapy. As in any line of work, health care providers range from excellent to subpar. Wide variation is found within the medical professions in terms of theory of approach, quality of care, and monetary concerns. Along with your participation, these factors influence the probability of your success.

No one intervention will work for everyone. Different health care providers see your neck or back pain in different ways based on their training, experience, and specialty. One therapist's idea of the right way to manage your pain may differ significantly from the approach of another therapist. If one period of rehab wasn't helpful, some other approach may be.

Unfortunately, disparity remains in the quality of therapy. Was the bulk of your care provided by the therapist or by an unlicensed tech who was trained on the job? Your therapist's hands are a valuable tool. Did they stretch, strengthen, and work on your spine or simply put a heat pack on it and massage the painful area? Did your program include exercises, stretches, and education on proper positioning, or were you in and out of the office in 30 minutes flat? A good therapy program needs time—time for you with the therapist to assess the problem, work through the treatment options, and learn what to do.

In reality, money influences your chances for success as much as clinical competence does. If you had therapy that wasn't helpful, what determined how long you received treatment? Was your program governed by an insurance program in which you saw the therapist once every few weeks or had an eight-visit limit? Did you stop attending after the first two weeks expecting to be better than you were? Many conditions respond well to a variety of treatment styles, and most improve steadily. If yours didn't, you should certainly ask why. Some conditions take months or years to evolve; assuming that a three- to four-week program will be long enough is not always reasonable. Perhaps your program hasn't helped only because you haven't been at it long enough.

There is no magic pill. To feel better, you have to do the work. Before you opt for surgery, confer with your doctor and ask yourself whether you've really committed to following your doctor's and therapist's recommendations. Only you know the answer.

COMMUNICATION AND TRUST

Communication between you and your physician is vital to getting the proper diagnosis and treatment and helping you decide whether to have surgery. After a treatment plan is suggested, you must make the final decision whether to go forward. The decision is yours, and you must be informed to make a good decision. The answers to the questions shown in figure 12.1 will help you make that decision. These questions help you evaluate the risks and potential complications of surgery versus the benefits. In addition, you will have realistic expectations of the outcome of the surgery. Some patients who have had severe problems such as significant weakness for months or years expect surgery to return all that they lost. Usually, surgery will only prevent progression and diminish associated pain. Some patients might have chosen not to have surgery had they known that it would not reverse all their problems, but other patients may not have recognized the severity of their condition. Communication is key.

Your surgeon should consider many factors before making a recommendation concerning surgery. The first consideration for your surgeon is to know what is not spine related. For instance, increasing numbness or weakness caused by neurological disease, such as multiple sclerosis, must be distinguished from numbness and weakness caused by spinal pathology. The surgeon is the last decision maker who can make this distinction before surgery.

1. What is the cause of my pain, numbness, or weakness?
2. What in my history, physical exam, and laboratory tests support that diagnosis?
3. What is your advice for treatment—surgery, medical, or other?
4. What are the risks and benefits of each kind of treatment?
5. What do you think is the best surgical approach to solve the problem?
6. What are the risks and complications of each approach and technique?
7. What are the benefits of this approach compared with others?
8. How much pain reduction or improvement should I expect?
9. Should we try alternative treatment first, such as injections or physical therapy?
10. What are the risks of waiting or delaying surgery? Is surgery urgent and, if so, why?
11. If this were your back, who would you ask for a second opinion?
12. How long will it be before I am walking, driving, going back to work, playing golf, and so forth?
13. How many surgeries like this have you done?
14. What team of doctors will evaluate me before, during, and after surgery?
15. What is the plan for postoperative care?
16. What alternative surgeries can be done?

Figure 12.1 Questions to ask your surgeon.

Second, the surgeon must qualify your personal risk factors and determine how they will influence your surgical outcome. Conditions such as diabetes or serious heart, kidney, or lung disease will affect the expectations of surgery.

Third, the surgeon should be aware of any psychological or social problems that might interfere with your postoperative care. Do you live alone? Do you have children? Do you have to walk up three flights of stairs? Have you experienced a recent death in the family?

Finally, your surgeon needs to know about the medications that you take. If you take opioid drugs such as hydrocodone, oxycodone, Percocet, or Dilaudid, be certain that your surgeon knows this. Don't forget other drugs, including alcohol. Alcohol withdrawal (delirium tremins) can cause confusion and combative behavior and may be life threatening in the postoperative period. Drug dependency produces extreme sensitivity to pain in the nerve ending. Additionally, exposure to strong molecules of morphine increases pain resistance. The doctor must know what substances your body is exposed to. If drug dependency is an issue, a proper detoxification program may produce better results than spinal surgery can. Sometimes spinal surgery is not fully effective until a detoxification program has been completed. Drug dependency is a frequent cause of failed surgery.

SURGICAL PLAN AND EXPECTATIONS

The surgeon must be able to explain in lay terms the proposed surgical plan and the reasons that the plan was chosen. This explanation not only provides a proper informed consent for surgery but also instills confidence in the patient about his or her ultimate recovery. A surgeon who cannot explain the surgical plan may not understand the plan or even have a plan. Results of spinal surgery are best when the plan is clear. Diagnostic tests should point clearly to the pathology. The experience of the surgeon allows her or him to pick the surgery that will correct the problem at the lowest risk. The surgeon should be well versed in multiple types of surgery, not just a few. For this reason, you may want to obtain a second opinion.

If the plan is performed as intended, you should experience a decrease in spinal pain or dysfunction. This expectation should be compared with the expectation if you did not have surgery. If surgery has a 70 percent chance of predominantly relieved symptoms and a 5 percent chance of worsening symptoms, you can make a satisfactory decision to have the surgery or not. You should ask the surgeon about his or her expectations, the probability of a certain postoperative condition, and the most probable outcome of the surgery. A surgeon may not necessarily know the exact outcome, but an experienced surgeon should be able to give you reasonably accurate answers to your questions.

Surgeons base their knowledge on a number of factors:

- Experience in operating on patients with similar conditions and operations
- Personal results and skills in doing that specific operation
- Statistical outcomes and expectations of other surgeons who perform this surgery

Be careful about how you respond to statistics. There are statistics, and then there are damned statistics. Consider your decision carefully based on all the information that you get from your surgeon. Be especially wary of any information that you find on the Internet. It is difficult, if not impossible, to know the veracity of information obtained from the Internet. Gather as many facts as possible from your surgeon and consider getting one good second opinion.

Trust must be developed between physician and patient, and certainly between surgeon and patient. You need to trust that your surgeon will not abandon you, that the surgeon will do everything possible after surgery to enhance recovery, and that the surgeon has picked the best operation for you under your circumstances. You must trust that the surgeon will carry out a continual plan for recovery. Complications and poor results can occur with the best surgical plans, the best intentions, and the best postoperative follow-up. Your surgeon should have a plan to deal with problems. Remember that your trust in your surgeon is of high importance.

Ask the "what if" questions: What if I still have symptoms? What if the symptoms return a year later? What if a complication develops? Communication is a vital component in the doctor–patient relationship, and this communication goes two ways. You must communicate properly all the causes and symptoms of your problems as best you can, as well as any feelings that you have about surgery, such as fear. The surgeon must communicate her or his understanding and clearly state the role that she or he will take in your medical condition.

Your surgeon needs to make sure that you understand the anatomy of your problem, the approach that the surgeon will use, and the techniques available to fix your problem.

Spinal Anatomy

Your surgeon should make sure that you have a basic grasp of spinal anatomy and that you understand his or her description of the surgical procedure. In order to understand your spinal surgeon, you should become familiar with the anatomy of the spine. You should understand terms that surgeons use, such as laminectomy and radiculopathy.

The spine is like a house. Feel the bones in the back of your neck and lower back. These bones, called the spinous process, are like the steeple of the house. The spinous process comes off the roof of the spine, which is called a lamina. Operations that refer to laminectomy remove the lamina, or roof. A laminotomy removes only part of the lamina. The spine is not solid bone; it is a mobile structure. Ligaments are found between the laminas at each level. The most common ligament in the roof of the spinal canal between the laminas is the yellow ligament ligamentum flavum. The walls of the house are made up of pillars, which are known as pedicles. The windows where the nerve exits the spinal cord to go into the arms or legs are called the foramen. The joints that attach one vertebra with the next are the facette joints. Think of the spine as a series of multiple joints. Each vertebra is numbered: C1, C2, C3, C4, C5, C6, and C7 are in the neck, and L1, L2, L3, L4, and L5 are in the lumbar region. Joints, intervertebral discs, and ligaments are between vertebrae. (For example, between the L4 vertebra and the L5 vertebra are the L4–L5 joint, the L4–L5 intervertebral disc, and the L4–L5 ligaments.) The floor of the house is made up of the vertebral bodies that the pillars attach to and the intervertebral discs. An intervertebral disc is a multilayered ligament that looks like a woven basket. It is laminated with multiple layers like belts on a truck tire. It attaches to the vertebrae above and below and allows motions between the vertebrae. Two facette joints behind the intervertebral disc make up a joint. L4–L5 has a disc and two facette joints. This joint has its own nerves. If it is sprained and injured, it hurts. The joint will swell and become inflamed like any other joint. The inside of the house is the spinal canal. The spinal cord is in the neck, and the cauda equina is in the back.

If the intervertebral disc develops a tear between its layers and its dense liquid center (nucleous pulposa) bulges out, a disc herniation has occurred. A fragment of the disc that extrudes into the spinal canal in the neck can be extremely dangerous and cause paralysis. More often, a combination of the disc bulge, a ligament buckling, and joint arthritis can seriously narrow the spinal canal, the living space for the spinal cord or cauda equina. A slow or sudden loss of strength, bladder control, and sensation may occur. This result constitutes a compelling reason for surgery.

The nerves run through the house, starting at the brain and extending all the way down to the bottom of the toes. The nerves help the surgeon pinpoint where the problem is in the spine, what nerve is involved, and what pathology is involved at that segment, based on the history and physical examination.

An additional factor to consider is the movement of the spine. The spine can flex, extend, bend laterally, and twist. These movements can change the relations of the spine anatomy. Anyone with back or neck pain knows that certain movements provoke or worsen the pain. We use this biomechanical function in the maneuvers of the physical exam to help diagnose the cause of your pain or symptoms. When you bend forward (flexion), the spinal canal and windows open and the nerves become taut. When you arch your neck or back backward (extension), the spinal canal closes, which squeezes the nerves, but the nerves relax. Patients have different symptom complexes, symptoms based on spinal motion that take into account these biomechanical factors. The surgeon's understanding of the anatomy of the spine and nerves and the biomechanical function of the spine allows her or him to pinpoint the source of your symptoms and design an operation to correct the problem.

Surgical Approach

Spine surgery has evolved considerably over the past 20 years thanks to key technical advances. You may be amazed that spine surgery has several approaches and techniques.

The surgical approach refers to how the surgeon enters through the skin into the spine. For example, the surgical approach to get to a disc is different from one used to correct a problem with the facette joints, spinous process, or vertebral body. The three main approaches are the posterior approach, the anterior approach, and the lateral approach.

Always ask your surgeon to describe the safest approach for your surgery. You may choose to get a second opinion or find a surgeon who is skilled in that approach. Not all surgeons have the same training.

Techniques

Each approach has a technique. The three techniques are microscopic, endoscopic, and loop-assisted direct vision. Ask your surgeon which technique he or she will use. The microscopic technique means that the surgeon will look through a microscope into the spine. Endoscopic surgery uses some type of visualization source, such as a fiber-optic cable, which is introduced into the wound. The surgery is performed as the surgeon looks at the monitor. The surgeon approaches through the foramen using an endoscope. The surgeon may choose a posterior approach into the floor of the spine using a microscope or an anterior approach through the chest into the spine using an endoscope. Loop-assisted direct vision is another technique. Ask the surgeon which technique he or she will use. Also, preoperative MRI scans or CAT scans can help with the localization of the problem, such as a herniated disc versus a tumor versus an aneurysm.

A new and exciting approach to surgery is image-aided computerized surgery. Multiple computer-generated pictures of your spine are produced in real time in the operating room while you are under anesthesia, allowing the surgeon to identify the abnormalities. The surgical instruments have sensors that produce a motion picture of the tool, such as a screw or probe, as it advances through your body into the abnormal area. This technique allows for extreme precision.

Nerve monitoring is often used to warn the surgeon that a nerve is being compromised or injured. This helps to save the nerve because it warns the surgeon that something may be going wrong. Also, monitoring of a nerve and removal of an obstruction may help the surgeon know that she or he has removed what was damaging or impairing the nerve and will confirm that the surgery was successful. Nerve monitoring can also help the surgeon know whether the surgical intervention will result in a full recovery.

Intraoperative nerve monitoring is an electrical monitoring of the nerves in the surgical area. This important, complicated procedure requires experience and communication between the neuro-monitoring technician and the surgeon. Your surgeon may be able to tell which nerves are abnormal at the start of the surgery, which ones improve or get worse during surgery, and what the nerve situation is after surgery. This technique is often helpful in complicated cases. Ask whether it is available.

YOUR SURGICAL TEAM

Always ask your surgeon who is on the team. We suggest that all surgeons cooperate with internal medicine specialists before the operation and with the anesthesia team during the surgery, use intraoperative nerve monitoring, if required, during surgery, and cooperate with nurses and doctors after surgery.

Does your surgeon have a team? Do the same people always make up the team? Have the lines of communication been established and perfected over time? This aspect is as important as the surgeon's experience and expertise.

TYPES OF SPINAL SURGERY

The three main types of surgeries are decompressive surgeries, spinal stabilization and fusion, and motion preservation techniques such as artificial discs.

Decompressive Surgeries

When abnormal tissues press on a nerve and produce pain, weakness, numbness, or neurological dysfunction, we can decompress them. When a disc herniation is pressing on the nerve, the surgery is called a discectomy, a removal of the portion of the disc pressing on the nerve. If the lamina or roof is pressing on the nerves, the surgery to be done is a laminectomy to remove the lamina or a laminotomy to remove part of the lamina. A partial facetectomy removes part of the joint that is pressing on the nerves. Decompressive operations are generally done to relieve leg or arm pain instead of back pain.

Spinal Stabilization and Fusion

These operations are designed to cure back or neck pain caused by movement. Spinal fusion surgery has been a godsend for patients whose decompression surgeries have failed. Scarred nerves, degenerated abnormal joints, misalignments of the vertebrae, slippage of the spine, and severe inflammatory conditions of intravertebral disc space may all cause severe pain when that joint is moved. Stopping that movement by an interbody fusion often gives the patient total relief.

Generally, operations designed to cure pain from the neck or back are designed to stop painful motion of the joint. The concept is that the severe pain caused by the movement of a joint can be eliminated if the motion in the joint can be stopped. Spinal fusions can be extremely successful in ending joint pain. The technique of the fusion is critical for producing a good long-term result.

The intervertebral disc is responsible for 80 percent of the biomechanical motion and activity in the joint. The facette joint is responsible for the additional 20 percent. The best way to stop the motion in a disc segment is to remove the intervertebral disc and replace it with bone or a bone-forming substance that allows bone to grow from one vertebra to another across the intervertebral disc. These procedures are referred to as interbody fusions, meaning fusions between the two vertebral bodies. Bone grows from one vertebral body across another.

Specific techniques are used to remove the discs and the joint to allow this fusion to take place. Bone-stimulating materials such as bone morphogenic protein promote this fusion by stimulating the cells for this bone to grow across the bridge. The patient's own bone, bone from a bone bank, bone morphogenic protein, or certain polymer substances such as PEAK or titanium can be used to enhance the fusion process. The delivery of these fusion-producing products to the disc space is a critical portion of the surgical technique and requires a good approach. The surgeon should use the approach that allows safe entry into the disc space without disturbing normal structures.

An additional component of the spinal fusion is the internal fixation—the screws, rods, and other mechanical devices that hold the two vertebra in place until the fusion is complete. Motion interferes with spinal fusion, so this hardware holds the spine rigidly or semirigidly to protect the fusion as it heals and the bone grows. The use of screws, such as pedicle screws, improves the fusion rate and makes it more likely that the fusion will be successful. But some controversy remains about using screws and rods in a patient's back. Some patients are reluctant to have hardware inserted into their spines. Some have had problems with spinal fusions and have attributed those complications to the screws that were placed in the back.

A common concern is that if you do one fusion, you will need to fuse the next level. Consider these factors.

- Anyone who has one bad segment is more likely than the average person to have another bad segment. Many patients have progressive degenerative disc disease that is affecting the entire spine. It often is impossible to prove that the spinal fusion caused an adjacent level to degenerate in a patient who had progressive degeneration over the entire spine. Imagine that you are 35 years old. If the amount of pain and disability resulting from one joint in the spine is severe enough to cause you major impairment in activity and you know that you might need additional surgery by age 55, would you choose to have a productive 20 years even if you may need surgery later?

- The method and technique of fusing one segment can influence whether another segment needs to be fused in the future. A joint fused in a bad position will place abnormal strain on the adjacent level. A joint fused in a crooked position will affect the other joints. In the spine, natural curves and motions are present. The lumbar spine and lower back have a normal, natural curve that allows proper positioning of the body when you lift materials over your head. When one segment is fused at a crooked angle, causing a loss of the natural lordosis, the result is kyphosis in the lumbar spine. This condition puts tremendous strain on adjacent levels and leads to premature disc degeneration at an adjacent level. Therefore, the techniques of the spinal fusion should enhance proper lumbar lordosis. For example, interbody fusions are better at correcting loss of proper lumbar lordosis and producing a proper position for the fusion. Pedicle screw fixation can hold the position at the time of the fusion until the fusion heals.

- The method of the spinal fusion should not directly injure the levels adjacent to the fusion. Therefore, the surgeon should avoid any approach or technique that injures the joint capsule or disc at the adjacent level. Reconstructive surgery of the spine involves motion preservation or artificial disc replacement. The same principles apply; the approach should be safe and effective and not cause additional problems. The technique used to insert the artificial disc is a major component in producing a good result, allowing the prosthesis to accomplish what it is designed to do.

- The mechanics and materials of the prosthesis are important. Is it made of polyethylene? Metal? Are the materials biocompatible? Has mechanical testing of the materials shown sufficient integrity to allow the prosthesis to last the required time? You should trust your physician and surgeon to choose the proper technique and materials. Feel free to discuss these choices with your surgeon. Figure 12.2 lists some questions that you will need your surgeon to answer before you decide to go ahead with fusion surgery or artificial disc replacement.

---

1. What are the surgeon's results with these techniques?
2. What approach to the spine will be used, and what is the surgeon's experience in that approach?
3. What materials will be used in the fusion or artificial disc replacement?
4. What is the preexisting spinal alignment? Is instability present?
5. What is the expected result for the disc adjacent to the segment proposed for surgery?
6. What is the current available scientific evidence that the proposed operation will be effective in my case, considering my existing condition of spinal alignment instability, source of pain, and presence of nerve root injury or irritation?

Figure 12.2   Questions regarding fusion surgery or artificial disc replacement.

Motion Preservation Techniques

The original idea behind artificial disc replacement was that the artificial disc would restore normal motion to the disc space and the preserved motion would prevent problems in adjacent levels. That is, the technique would better preserve the disc above and the disc below.

In the United States in recent years, artificial disc replacement has proved to be as effective as spinal fusion and allows a quicker return to activity. As with any medical intervention, artificial disc replacement has pros and cons. On the pro side, an artificial disc can restore normal motion to the disc space. Preserving motion prevents problems to the joints above and below the affected disc. In a fusion, the joints above and below the fusion take on the stress of the fused joint and later could become problems. The artificial joint may prevent that from occurring.

On the con side, determining the normal motion for a specific patient can be difficult. The patient's body may establish that parameter postoperatively. Questions also arise about whether the artificial joint will prevent problems to the adjacent joints. Some patients develop progressive multilevel degenerative disc disease that is not remedied by the operation. Finally, good artificial disc replacement requires that there not be a major slippage, instability, or abnormal position of the two joints to be connected. Abnormal position or slippage causes excessive wear and tear on the metal and plastic components of the prosthesis, resulting in higher instances of misalignment, spondylolisthesis, or bad positioning of the two segments to be fused.

IS SURGERY FOR YOU?

The decision to have surgery is critical. You need to make your decision based on all the information that you get from your surgeon. Compelling reasons may support the decision to have surgery, but you may wish to try other treatments first. If those treatments fail and symptoms persist, surgery may be the only alternative, a strong indication for surgery. Relative indications are those that don't necessitate surgery, but you might choose surgery to preserve your lifestyle. Consider whether the benefits outweigh the risks.

To make this decision, communication with your doctor, surgeon, or neuro-orthopedist is critical. You must understand the exact origin of your symptoms based on your history, exam, and tests (HELP). Consider your doctor's prescription, medical versus surgery. The urgency depends on the cause. Waiting too long can have consequences, as can rushing in.

When surgery is the prescription, assess your surgeon's experience and abilities. Ask relevant questions and carefully consider the answers. With your surgeon, choose the proper technique and approach to maximize the probability of a favorable outcome and minimize complications. The team approach pre- and postoperation can make all the difference. Trust in your doctor is an essential element. Will he or she always be there for you?

The art of surgery is more than just cutting. It is knowing when to act and when to wait through careful evaluation and communication with the patient.

Index

NOTE: Page numbers followed by an italicized *f* or *t* indicate that there is a figure or table on that page, respectively.

About the Authors

Vincent Fortanasce, MD, is clinical and associate professor of neurology at the University of Southern California in the departments of neurology and physical therapy. He is ranked as one of the best medical specialists in North America and has treated such high-profile individuals as Pope John Paul II and Major League Baseball Hall of Famer Tommy Lasorda. Over nearly four decades, Dr. Fortanasce has treated Olympic and professional athletes as a world-renowned neurologist, neuro-orthopedist, and rehabilitation specialist. He has appeared as a medical expert on *60 Minutes*, *The Today Show*, *Dr. Phil*, *Dateline*, CNN's *Paula Zahn Now*, *Hard Ball with Chris Mathews*, XM satellite radio,

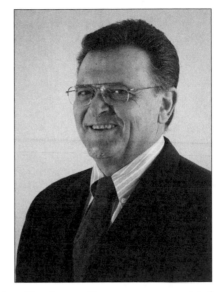

and scores of national and local television and radio shows. Fortanasce was chief of neuro-orthopedics at Rancho Los Amigos Hospital at USC and neurological consultant to the spine centers at St. Vincent Medical Center and Casa Colina Hospital. He has been quoted in the *New York Times*, *Sports Illustrated*, *USA Today*, *U.S. News & World Report*, *Time* magazine, and many other prestigious publications. He also hosts his own syndicated radio program, *St. Joseph's Radio Presents*.

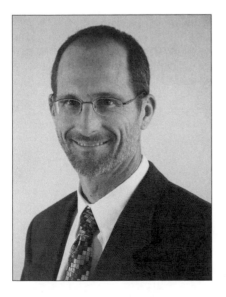

David Gutkind, DPT, is a doctor of physical therapy and an orthopedic clinical specialist. During his professional career, he has specialized in ergonomics as a treatment intervention for both the cause and prevention of musculoskeletal injury to the spine. He has taught ergonomics at the university level, provided on-site training programs that emphasize spinal care and injury prevention at the corporate level, and conducted hundreds of individual and group training classes on lifting and body mechanics techniques. Gutkind lives in Southern California and continues to practice orthopedic physical therapy along with ergonomic instruction.

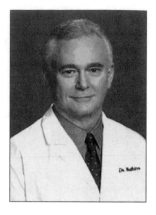

Robert Watkins, MD, is a spine surgeon and codirector of the Marina Spine Center at Marina Hospital in Marina del Rey, California. He is the former chief of spinal surgery at USC. His expertise ranges from innovative spine surgeries to treatment of sport-related injuries. In his practice, he treats collegiate, professional, and Olympic athletes across the United States. He has served more than 25 years as a spine consultant to the Los Angeles Dodgers, the Los Angeles Kings, the Los Angeles Angels, the Los Angeles Lakers, the Anaheim Mighty Ducks, and golfers on the PGA Tour. He has extensive experience in spinal surgery and postoperative rehabilitation of professional athletes, returning most athletes to full performance. As a surgeon, he has participated in more than 11,000 spine surgeries in a career that has spanned 30 years, and he currently completes nearly 250 surgeries a year. He has also developed an extensive coordinated core nonoperative program of rehabilitation without surgery.

You'll find other outstanding fitness resources at

www.HumanKinetics.com/fitnessandhealth

In the U.S. call 1-800-747-4457

Australia 08 8372 0999 • Canada 1-800-465-7301
Europe +44 (0) 113 255 5665 • New Zealand 0800 222 062

HUMAN KINETICS
The Premier Publisher for Sports & Fitness
P.O. Box 5076 • Champaign, IL 61825-5076 USA

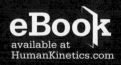

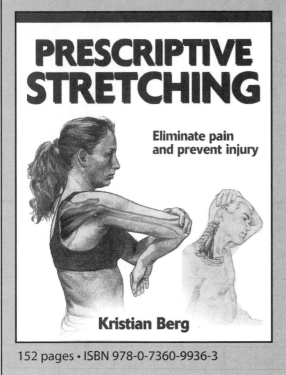
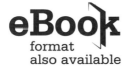